Addressing Health Inequalities through Community Media

Fazal Malik

Addressing Health Inequalities through Community Media

The Transformative Power of Voice and Agency

palgrave
macmillan

Fazal Malik
Amity University
Dubai, United Arab Emirates

ISBN 978-3-031-35236-2   ISBN 978-3-031-35237-9 (eBook)
https://doi.org/10.1007/978-3-031-35237-9

This Palgrave Macmillan imprint is published by the registered company Springer Nature Switzerland AG.
The registered company address is: Gewerbestrasse 11, 6330 Cham, Switzerland

This book is dedicated to all those who strive to amplify stifled voices and validate alternative ways of knowing and doing things

Acknowledgements

This study has immensely benefited from the lives and worldviews of the listeners, volunteers and participants of Community Radio Stations in Nottingham. This work is indebted to their experiences.

A special thank you goes to Prof. Roger Bromley, Prof. Patrick Williams, Prof. Parvati Raghuram, and Dr Musharaf Hussain OBE and the Specialist Health Promotion Team of then Nottingham Primary Care Trust.

This project would not have been possible without the support of my wife, Ruby, and our children, Nibras and Rayyan. Their critique of my work helped me reflect on my own politics and practice.

Contents

Chapter 1
Introduction

Exploring the role marginalized peoples' cultural practices and experiential knowledge can play in their fight against social exclusion, the book contextualises insights from a community radio station in knowing alternative ways of knowing and doing things. Looking specifically at the efforts of the marginalized communities to address the issues emanating from the inequalities in health, the study, carried out over two decades ago in the city of Nottingham, becomes critically important today to understand the disproportionate impact of Coivid-19 pandemic on the most vulnerable groups, especially the ethnic, racial and immigrant communities. These communities, historically living in the deprived areas of the post-industrialized cities in the UK, are roped in cycle of poverty. The latest 2021 census in the UK, while recording increase in the number of Muslim population, shows that 39 per cent of this population lives in the most underprivileged areas of England and Wales. Caught up in the cycle of deprivation and disadvantage, members of this community, as high risk group, live with the 'worst health outcomes' in comparison with 'all social group and ethnicities' in the UK (Sufyan, 2022).

Though the policy frameworks and regulations put emphasis to understand public health within the context of lived experiences of people, the Covid-19 Pandemic has demonstrated that policy frameworks and pledges remain far from reality while the inequalities continue to impact health and wellbeing of millions of people. In many parts of the developed world, including the UK, the socio-economic disadvantages along with racism continue to define ethnic and racial disparities in many post-industrial cities. As per the report[1] *Ethnicity and outcomes from covid-19* by the Intensive Care National Audit Research Centre (ICNARC) UK, 34 percent of the critically ill patients due to covid-19 infection were from black, Asian or minority ethnic groups in mid 2020. Similarly, Public Health England puts the mortality from people form minority ethnic groups due to covid-19 two times higher than their white counterparts.

The disproportionate impact of Covid 19 on the health of ethnic minorities in the UK is also being linked to the 'cultural and structural racism' seen on rise in the

F. Malik, *Addressing Health Inequalities through Community Media*,
https://doi.org/10.1007/978-3-031-35237-9_1

many western societies. Though the impact of racism on health has been investigated from a range of perspectives (Williams, 2012, Public Health England 2020), how it affects the health of the people of Black and South Asian origin in the UK in the current Covid-19 pandemic shows the deep rooted discrimination and racial prejudice that define public services in modern societies. Taking notice of the risk of exposure to Covid-19 and effect of inequality on response to the infection, Nielsen & Albertsen (2023) argue for prioritizing healthcare that can provide 'weight to protecting the socially disadvantaged'. In their 'ex-ante' and 'ex-post' discourse, the authors draw support from the global mortality figures from the Covid-19 to make a case to sensitize needs for supporting those who are socially and economically disadvantaged. Taking cognizance of the 'generic fairness argument for the claim that welfare states' make, the authors argue that 'it is not fair to when disadvantaged people suffer more from the danger of exposer as well as the impact of the pandemic. Besides the social and economic disadvantage, impact of racism and social determinants of health, including discrimination and prejudices lead to chronic diseases and lower life expectancy among the people living on the margins of the society. While the consequences of health inequalities are known and there is a fund of empirical and conceptual literature available to understand explore what this disparity can lead to, the latest evidence of the health inequalities illustrated by the Covid-19 urgently seeks solutions by better understanding and addressing the causes of this inequity in health outcomes of ethnic minority groups.

Against this backdrop, the study, influenced by the contemporary desire for more pluralistic and egalitarian practices in fight against inequalities and injustices, brings together perspectives and practices to challenge the presumed universality of Western knowledge one hand and on the other examines the possibilities of alternative ways of addressing inequalities. In this effort, the book using a case study, demonstrates that how a faith-based community broadcasting initiative can be an empowering platform for communicative interaction for the people to engage, reflect and organize. The case study of Radio Ramzan[2] in Nottingham operated during the month of Ramadan of the Islamic calendar provided a context to the spiritual life of the members of the Mirpuri[3] community, who experience a range of socio-economic disadvantages, especially inequalities in health and wellbeing. Within this discourse, the book, at length, engages with the worldviews of the people whose cultural identity and socio-economic status mark them as minorities and who are left out in a commercial and largely biased media discourse. Exploring the agency through participatory action research, the study examines how peoples' reference to cultural practices and experiential knowledge can empower them to counter their situated and essentialized existence. This existence, defined by higher unemployment, low educational achievements, poor housing and especially inequalities in health, marginalise many communities in poor neighbourhoods. In in absence of voice, time and again, this 'existence' is 'othered' and often stigmatised.

Research suggests that whether measured in terms of mortality, life expectancy or health status, inequalities in health in the UK is a fact, making it one of the most unequal societies in the developed world. Along with low achievement in education, higher unemployment, poor housing and higher rate of crime, poor health is also disproportionately prevalent among minority ethnic groups. When seen in combination with racism and discrimination, the racial background of people is seen contributing to the illness (McKenzie, 2003). However, the relationship between health and ethnicity is not a simple one. Like any other group living in poor neighbourhoods, the white population in these areas shares the inequalities in health but there is a clear and direct link between the health of people and the area they live in. It is, thus, not surprising to observe that the health and wellbeing of minority ethnic and racial groups, mostly living in inner city areas of the post-industrial towns in the UK, show health inequalities especially in coronary heart diseases, obesity and diabetes.

Caught-up in a vicious circle of social exclusion, and economic disadvantage, this burden is further aggravated by cultural isolation, structural racism and discrimination, affecting both physical and mental health of these people. There is a fund of literature available to demonstrate the impact of poor housing, unemployment, low educational attainment on health and wellbeing, but all interventions and efforts to address these health inequalities emerge from the top to bottom socio-scientific approach that ignores the cultural and living realities of the victims of these inequalities. Besides the structural issues which are manifest in a number of social and economic inequalities, there is a growing body of evidence which suggests many cultural reasons including stigmatization, racism and discriminations which directly contribute to health inequalities (Byrene et al., 2020).

A unique feature of the book is how it theorizes disadvantage in the inner city pockets of the UK by juxtaposing it with the 'third world[4]' narrative of modernization which still resonates in many parts of the developing world. By looking at the geographic and cultural roots of those living in poor urban areas of post-industrial UK, the book forcefully argues how the consequences of 'victim-blaming' and top to bottom interventions in both developing and developed world leads to powerlessness.

The book engages with a unique methodological approach adopted to critique the dominant way of 'being human' and validate subaltern knowledge and experience. This methodological uniqueness informed by various emancipatory and critical perspectives including feminism, poststructuralism and liberation theology goes beyond conventional silos to develop a non-essentialist approach to understand the issues of participation and empowerment. These perspectives are contextualized within communication studies, human geography and cultural studies to provide a dynamic framework to analyze the field study outside the conventional rigidities and academic silos. Offering unique insights into the growing interdisciplinary scholarship about place, media and health, it brings in fresh perspectives into social disadvantage within the inner city pockets of the UK by engaging with the debates emerging from the margins. This way, the book articulates for decentering the power in order to allow people from peripheries to assert and find their own ways to deal with the inequalities they face.

In the Chap. 2, tone is set by contextualizing the research questions within the academic discourse to examine the socio-scientific basis of the modernization paradigm, foreground marginal worldviews, and to examine the role of cultural practices in addressing the issues of powerlessness. The chapter draws parallels between the discourses of developmentalism and social inclusion to illustrate the influence of Western knowledge and its principles, especially that of modernization as a process and ideology in constructing the 'Third World' and the 'Inner city'. This analogy, supported through a thorough review of literature, reveals the links between the politics of aid in the 'Third world' and the discourse of urban regeneration in the 'first world'. The chapter looks ahead to find the ways and means within the participatory and liberatory movements to re-conceptualize these constructs within the worldviews of marginalized people and their cultural practices to increase community participation in fighting inequalities.

Chapter 3 conceptualizes a dynamic multi-perspective and an interdisciplinary framework to examine the fieldwork. The methodology chapter becomes very critical in articulating epistemological plurality and understanding the multiplicity of subject positions especially when the focus is on emancipation from all levels of oppression and inequalities. So, this methodology is influenced by several critical, emancipatory and liberation theology perspectives, sharing its politics with many contemporary movements like women's, environment, 'Third World', human rights, anti-racism, anti-capitalism and anti-war campaigns. This framework influenced by the practice of experiential and contextual learning facilitates a more democratic relationship between the knower and known and rejects false dualisms. The chapter goes on to problematize my position (researcher) within the project to understand how this position affects the research, and in turn, gets affected by it.

The Chap. 4 problematizes the concept of community to move away from the fixed understanding of the community and embrace a more positional construct of community. This is also important as the study assesses the role of the community radio station in facilitating communicative interaction. So to fully engage with the community platform, this chapter Juxtaposes various strategic conceptions and problematizes the fixed notion of community to examine the expanded consciousness of the people in their egalitarian participation in the project. The chapter looks into the heterogeneities and diversities within the concept and unpacks the political, geographic, populist, communal and communitarian concepts of community. This analysis is in sync with the overall theme and politics of this book.

In Chap. 5 analysis is carried out of the situated dealings of health and wellbeing of the people living in inner-city areas to uncover the discursively constructed 'managerial' policies and practices of health services in the UK. The chapter examines the narrow clinical understanding of health and wellbeing in the most of the epidemiological work fails to engage with the cultural and political aspects of life. It fails to appreciate the knowledge and experience of the people living on the margins. The chapter thus engages with the debate on the racialization of health assesses the discourse of healthism on one hand and on the other challenges the fixed notion of inequality. The chapter, following on the critiques the process of medicalization of health inequalities and argues for a holistic approach to health and well-being where the cultural practices and experiences of the victims of health inequalities becoming part of the discourse in fighting exclusion.

Chapter 6 puts all the arguments, made in previous chapters, to an analysis through the case study of the faith bases radio station in Nottingham. The case study, using participatory research, evaluate the relationship between faith, place and media to find out if and how locally owned and operated radio station can offer a medium of validating alternative visions of participation, power and action. A month-long, multi-agency, Health Education Awareness Project (HEAP), conceived and delivered through the local radio station, is used to test how a community-based approach can offer an equitable and effective approach in dealing with inequalities in health.

The Chap. 7 maps the key themes emerging at the intersection of agency, identity and social mobility. With community radio providing a context, the framework developed by bringing together the feminist, poststructuralist and liberation theology perspectives is used to raise critical consciousness about the causes and consequences of marginalization on one hand and on the other explore the possibilities of dealing with it. The chapter engages with the solidarities and identities which came to the forefront as the community radio provided a common frame of reference for the people who share common interests in terms of faith, country of origin and kinship on the one hand, and on the other are grouped, uncritically, as Asians, immigrants, non-white, disadvantaged, and so on through the discourses associated with bureaucracies, popular media, politics and academia.

At the end, the book goes back where it started; the Covid-19 pandemic and how it exposes the grotesque inequalities that still define life in many pockets of the western world. The epilogue of the book engages with the renewed debate on health inequalities and provides some insights into how health inequalities can be reduced.

Notes

1. Ethnicity and outcomes from covid-19: The isaric CCP-UK prospective observational cohort study of hospitalized patients, 3 June 2020, GOV.UK Available at: https://www.gov.uk/government/publications/ethnicity-and-outcomes-from-covid-19-the-isaric-ccp-uk-prospective-observational-cohort-study-of-hospitalised-patients-3-june-2020 (Accessed: September 18, 2022).
2. The station is named Radio Ramzan (Urdu version of Ramadan) to give it a South Asian flavour, where the Arabic letter (ض) 'Da' is mostly pronounced with the 'Z' sound while in the Arab world this letter is pronounced with 'D' sound. For the sake of authenticity, the author uses Ramzan for Radio and Ramadan for the month of fasting.
3. Mirpuris are the people who originate from the Mirpuri district of 'Pakistan Administered Kashmir'. This part was culturally and linguistically part of the pre-partition Punjab, but geo- politically it has been a part of the Princely State of Jammu and Kashmir – an autonomous entity under the British Raj. After the British left, and the subcontinent was partitioned into India and Pakistan along communal lines, Jammu and Kashmir, got divided

between two newborn countries, and have fought few wars on the issue which is a highly complex and contentious one, and it is beyond the scope of this thesis to explore these complexities (For a detailed discussion on the Kashmir problem, see Lamb, 2003; Schofield, 1996; Ganguly, 1997). The immigration pattern of people from Mirpur is well documented (Dayha, 1974; Ballard, 1991). Mirpuris have been working with the British merchant navy since before the Second World War. During the war, these people worked in South Shields, where they facilitated the arrival of more from their villages. After the war, British factories- mainly cotton industries- needed manpower, and Mirpuris fulfilled this demand. Ballard (1991) believes this was the start of the chain-migration as large numbers of relations and friends joined them in the UK. Later, the World Bank financed Mangla Dam in the heart of Mirpur, which displaced thousands of people who used the compensation money to immigrate to Britain. After settling down in the UK, flows of remittances back to the villages of origin encouraged more to come. Mirpuris make up the largest group of Muslim living in the UK.

4. Labeling and terminology is problematic in the development discourse. The term 'Third World' has evolved historically. In the current context, the term is used is used to refer to industrially and technologically less developed countries in Asia, Africa and Latin America. Although the economic and technological situations in some of these countries have changed the labels have not. The use of 'Third World; and 'First World' in this thesis is deliberate to highlight the binary divisions created by modernism which still continue to dominate academic discourses. The thesis, however, does not subscribe to this classification and throughout this thesis, keeps these labels within inverted commas.

Chapter 2
Marginalized Worldviews

A run through the literature on issues surrounding social exclusion in the 'first world' (Levitas, 1999; Hardill et al., 2001) and the debate on the developmentalism in the 'Third-World' (Golding, 1974; Rogers, 1976; Escobar, 1992) shows interesting similarities. Both talk about the poor, though there is a change in the lexicon: in the backyards of the West, poverty has been replaced by exclusion, development by inclusion and intervention by partnership. No doubt, the poverty in the West is different from poverty in the East, but in both situations the consequences of poverty remain the same: powerlessness.

Both these discourses have been criticised for adopting the top- down and centralised managerial approach, and having a socio-scientific bias along with a contextual bankruptcy (Gutierrez, 1988; Nandy, 1992; Escobar, 1995a, b). The discourse of social exclusion is seen to be the continuation of the modernisation inspired developmentalism project (Hardill et al., 2001). In both discourses, the superiority of the Western knowledge dwarfs the knowledge and experience of disadvantaged people. Another striking feature of this comparison is the fact that the majority of people caught in the circle of social exclusion in the West have a direct link with the areas in Pakistan, India and Bangladesh, which have been the focus of relentless developmentalism practiced by Western governments, development agencies and non- governmental organizations. Some scholars see the 'Third World' being produced, managed and organised by the powerful countries and institutions for ideological and political-economic motives (Esteva, 1992; Crush, 1995). Similarly, the discourse of social exclusion is seen to be managed by bureaucracies and regimes to problematise 'otherness' and abnormalize spaces (Levitas, 1998; Shah, 1998). In the context of poverty in the 'Third World', the following definition of poverty by the 1995 Copenhagen World Summit on Social Development, sums up this dispossession:

> *Lack of income and productive resources to ensure sustainable livelihoods; hunger and malnutrition; ill health; limited or lack of access to education and other basic services;*

F. Malik, *Addressing Health Inequalities through Community Media*,
https://doi.org/10.1007/978-3-031-35237-9_2

increased morbidity and mortality from illness; homelessness and inadequate housing; unsafe environments and social discrimination and exclusion. (IISD, 1995:57)

It is also characterised by lack of participation in decision-making and in civil, social and cultural life. (IISD, 1995:57). This definition holds good not only for the villages in the 'Third World' but can be applied to any inner city area in the first world, where many people live marginalized lives. In the UK, migrant communities inhabit some of the most deprived inner city areas. These spaces are characterised by poor health, poor housing, higher unemployment and low educational attainments, increased discrimination and racism (Nazroo, 1997; Werbner & Modood, 1997; Macpherson report, 1999; Abbas, 2005). While these conditions may not contribute to absolute poverty, a condition characterized by severe deprivation of basic human needs (IISD, 1995:57). In the UK many neighbourhoods can easily fit into this category as generations of people live in the areas which score very low on 'minimum acceptance of life'. The Social Exclusion Unit (SEU) of the government accepts the disproportionate representation of people from minority ethnic groups in poor urban areas:

People from minority ethnic communities are disproportionately represented in deprived areas. Fifty-six per cent live in the 44 most deprived local authorities in the country. And those 44 most deprived local authority areas contain proportionately four times as many people from minority ethnic groups as other areas. (SEU June, 2000)

As per the Joseph Rowntree Foundation, by the end of 1999 a quarter (26 per cent) of the British population was living in relative poverty. The study suggests that Britain now is the most unequal country in the developed world after New Zealand, with a wealth gap between the richest and poorest in society wider than in Ethiopia or Ghana (JRF, 2000). The 2001 Census figures show that there are about 1.8 million Muslims living in Britain. Although, the Muslim community in the UK is very diverse, representing various lingual, ethnic and racial backgrounds, over two thirds of this population originates from the Indian sub-continent. More than fifty per cent of British Muslims are born in Britain and a similar proportion is aged less than 25 years. The Muslim Council of Britain[1] (MCB), an umbrella organization of various mosques and Islamic institutions, quoting various government figures, says that the Muslim population has a poorer than average socio-economic profile with many people living in some of the most deprived areas. Their housing conditions, health indicators and educational attainments are considerably below national averages. The number of Muslims in the prison population is proportionately thrice their numbers in relation to the national population. These disadvantages lead to 'alienation and social exclusion' (MCB, 2003).

Tahir Abbas (2005:13) finds the government policies towards Muslim communities in the UK 'at best inconsistent, at worst patchy' when it comes to addressing issues in employment, housing and health. He, however, acknowledges some 'positives' within the race equality policy and practice like the provisions for Halal (Permissible) meals and permission for wearing Hijab (headscarf), but admits that members of Muslim communities remain disadvantaged at the local, regional and national level.

While the policy and strategies of governments fail to address the issues related to economic deprivation and social exclusion, in many instances, the state and its apparatuses blame victims rather than their own policies for this failure. The rhetoric of social exclusion/inclusion in the inner city areas of UK in many instances follows the pattern of 'ghetto formation' in the black neighbourhoods in the USA as reported by former US senator and sociologist Daniel Patrick Moynihan (Moynihan, 1965). This report highlighted how the causes of poverty were being attributed to the behaviour and cultural practices of the poor and not the social factors people live in (Williams, 1976). In the built up areas in Birmingham, Bradford, London and many small towns in the UK, where minority ethnic people live both as geographic communities and the communities of interest, the discourses of social exclusion 'problematise' and 'abnormalise' people and the spaces they live in. This is followed by creating regimes of bureaucracies to 'solve' problems and 'normalize' deviations (Levitas, 1998; Shah, 1998). This is not very different from what aid agencies, non-governmental and government organizations did decades ago in poor parts of the world. The cultural practices, beliefs and customs of the poor were held responsible for 'their plight' (Sachs, 1990; Escobar, 1992, 1995a, b).

Although there is not enough literature available on the comparisons and contrasts, efforts have been made to find common theoretical perspectives between the discourse of development in the 'Third World' and the discourse of social exclusion in the first world. International Development Studies at the University of Sussex first looked at this possibility when a seminar was organised in 1997 to explore 'insights from the South that can enrich debate in the North'.

The seminar concluded that whether you call it 'poverty' or 'social exclusion', the debate on deprivation was entering new territory, bringing in issues like access, personal security, vulnerability and self-esteem on the agenda in both North and South. The seminar also took note of the fact that there was a convergence in theory and practice between the North and the South, and globalisation was facilitating these connections. The seminar also highlighted the worries about groups who might find themselves marginalized in a society where others set the conditions for inclusion (O'Brien et al., 1997).

No doubt, with the gap between rich and poor widening in the West and many sections of the society being increasingly marginalized, the debate is entering new areas. But many scholars in the West are of the opinion that not much has been learnt from the failed development project, as many policies and schemes for fighting social exclusion are thought to show the same socio-scientific rationale of economic betterment as was obvious in the modernisation led developmentalism process. Ruth Levitas sees social exclusion reflecting a 'new Durkheimian hegemony' in which the poverty and disadvantage is seen a 'pathological deviation' from what is assumed to be 'essentially a fair social organisation' (Levitas, 1999: 211).

Since the Labour Party came to power in 1997, many policies and schemes have been formulated to end 'Inner city deprivation'. In fact, the inner city has become the target of endless programmes and strategies. Through rhetorical political debate on the issue, New Labour has created huge bureaucracies and an industry has now developed that promises to help the new poor'. But this discourse is not new. As the debate on developmentalism shows, the business-like approach in dealing with the poor and poverty has always taken the initiative away from victims and given it to politicians and technocrats. After the communal rioting in some northern towns of England in the autumn of 2001, the government commissioned an inquiry into the causes of these disturbances, which reported that government efforts to tackle the issues of social deprivation were disorganised, repetitive and often led to 'institutionalisation of problems'.

Unfortunately, the programmes devised to tackle the needs of many disadvantaged and disaffected groups, whilst being well intentioned and sometimes inspirational, often seemed to institutionalize the problems. The plethora of initiatives and programmes, with their baffling array of outcomes, boundaries, timescales and other conditions, seemed to ensure divisiveness and a perception of unfairness in virtually every section of the communities we visited (Cantle Report, 2001). This repetitive and muddled approach in addressing issues related to poverty is nothing new. There's a fund of literature available about the critique of the centralised approaches of dealing with the issues of 'underdevelopment' in poor countries of the world. But the following explanation by Escobar (1995a, b) written in the context of the 'Third World', sums up the current discourse of social exclusion in the UK:

> *... everywhere one looked, one found the busy, repetitive reality of development: government designing ambitious development plans, institutions carrying out development programmes in cities and countryside alike, experts studying development problems and producing theories ad nauseam, foreign experts everywhere, and development colonised reality, it became a reality.* (Escobar, 1995a, b:225)

Traditionally, the debate on development has remained confined to the 'Third World'. A quick run though the literature shows that development discourse has essentially been associated with the poverty beyond the shores of Western Europe and North America. While the —experts and expertise 'to deal with this poverty was emerging from the West, most of the —poor and poverty' was somewhere else. But with the emergence of the deprived inner city pockets, inhabited disproportionately by people of non-white and minority ethnic origin, surrounded by affluent suburbs, the poverty and social exclusion looks real. The class division and inequality are nothing new to the West, but with the spatalisation of poverty, the problem is more topical and immediate now. For instance, the literacy rates, health statistics, crime, unemployment figures, housing conditions, leisure and community services, dependence on social security among some of minority ethnic groups living in inner city areas in the UK (Nazroo, 1997; Modood, 1997) are as dramatic as among the people living in the slums and villages of many poor countries in the world. The situation for people living as minorities in the inner city areas of the West is further compounded by discrimination and racism, which is now being acknowledged to be institutional as well (MacPherson, 1999).

Due to the combination of these factors, many people belonging to minority ethnic groups feel excluded and alienated from the mainstream. The electoral data from Nottingham shows this disillusionment on the increase, as the turnout figures in the City elections fell considerably from an average of 46.6 percent in 1991 to 35 percent in 1995, to just 25.4 per cent in 2000 (Poverty in Nottingham, 2001). The figures for 1997 have been discounted due to the significant skew caused by the General Election. Although the election turnout is not an absolute yardstick to judge alienation and exclusion, it indicates the lack of participation in public life and decision making at the local level. The low turnout was observed higher in the areas inhabited by the members of minority ethnic groups. For example, Lenton with highest Muslim population in Nottingham showed a decline in turn out to 12.2 percent in 2000 from 36.6 percent in 1991. These figures clearly indicate that all areas experienced a considerable decline in the numbers of people who voted, but this decline is more profound in Lenton, with the higher concentration of people belonging to minority ethnic groups, especially the members of the Mirpuri community. These areas are also among the most deprived areas in the city. Another striking feature of the areas with high proportions of ethnic minority communities is that these areas also record high levels of racially aggravated crime. According to the Nottinghamshire Police (2000) the number of such incidents is on the increase in Forest and Radford areas, but more worrying is the fact that areas with relatively lesser concentration of such minorities also show an upward trend in recorded cases of racism. This is seen to increase the sense of exclusion and fear amongst minority ethnic groups in these neighbourhoods.

Before we go into the details of the discourse of social exclusion, let us first engage with the debate on developmentalism which is thought to have influenced the social policies in the deprived pockets of the West.

Modernisation and Developmentalism

Development discourse, or developmentalism, traditionally associated with the process of modernisation, has been unable to engage with the non-material aspects of human need. The dependence on Western knowledge, mostly scientific, has largely ignored the perspectives of marginalized groups in this discourse. Many scholars share the critical stance against established scientific knowledge, interest in local autonomy, culture and knowledge and the defense of localised, pluralistic grass roots movements (Esteva, 1987; Kothari, 1998; Sachs, 1990, Escobar, 1995a, b).

Different theories, standpoints and scholarships have also been associated with this journey of developmentalism since 1945. These arguments, borrowed from a wide range of disciplines, have been used to support, scrutinise and oppose the concept and process of development at different stages of its journey. In the process, development studies, cutting across the disciplinary boundaries, has created its own set of theories. The most significant concept that defined development for over five decades is that of modernisation. Theories associated with modernisation came to be known as the dominant paradigm, which still preoccupies most of the debate on development, though some scholars think this paradigm has passed. Modernisation is based on the neo-classical economic theory promoting and supporting the capitalist mode of production.

As an influential paradigm, with far reaching consequences, modernisation as a set of theories and concepts has its beginning in the evolutionary explanation of social change (Giddens, 1991). It has been used to create the development model for the 'Third World' countries, articulating a common set of assumptions about the nature of Western society and its ability to change a non-Western world which is considered 'deficient' both materially and culturally (Latham, 2000). Historically, there is a vast amount of literature available on development and the various arguments that surround this discourse (Lerner, 1958; Schramm, 1964; Rogers, 1976). Since the emergence of multi-lateral development assistance after the Second World War, we have seen the concept of 'Third Worldism' grow in the decade of the 1950s, followed by the period of great optimism in the sixties, which was defined by centralised economic planning, and the dominance of powerful mass media. The decade of the seventies is largely seen as a period of pessimism, as the debate on underdevelopment and exploitation started the critique of the dominant paradigm. This period also saw counter arguments gaining currency. Peoples' participation, women' role and basic needs became more important for the voiceless poor than capital-intensive technology and powerful channels of mass media. The decade of the 80 s is considered as a lost decade of development in which global recession brought problems in both poor and richer countries.

From 1990 onwards, a new shift and focus on development emerged. Sustainability and environmental protection, human rights and social welfare entered into development debate in a big way, emphasising the need for the people-centred participatory approaches, using critical consciousness and empowerment strategies in the process of development. This decade also marked the trend towards the globalisation of media, fashion and lifestyles, along with increased migration of people. Emerging from the West after World War II, modernization theory saw the modern nation resembling 'Western industrialized nation in all areas of society, including political, economic behavior and institutions, attitudes towards technology and science, and cultural mores' (Melkote & Steeves, 2001: 100). In many ways, development within the dominant paradigm meant development initiated, inspired and influenced by modernisation as a socio-economic process to influence change through scientific and technological innovation, increased industrialized production, mass consumption and rapid urbanization. In the course of time, modernisation has become a discourse- a set of words, symbols and processes that have supported all other structures and processes of promoting the Western concept of social change. It is seen as more than an economic theory and model of social evolution as the shift from religious to secular ideologies and transition from subsistence to technology-intensive economies are believed to be brought about through modernisation (Tipps, 1973).

As a process that encompasses overlapping concepts of westernization, rationalization and development, modernisation is 'reflected in – and reflective of – discourse, ideology and culture with a goal of replacing non-Western ideological, cultural' and even language system with Western systems; in essence' reshaping the reality of the people in the 'Third World' (Melkote & Steeves, 2001: 91–92). It promoted and supported economic development based on neo- classical economic theory, thus served as a vehicle for capitalist market economy. Since modernisation is often associated with economic development, and many earlier proponents of modernisation saw it as incompatible with the traditions and customs of people. These scholars thought that breaking from the traditions was a prerequisite to economic progress. Using the economic system, Rostow (1960), identified sequential and linear stages as the pathway to modernisation. Others went further to link modernisation and economic 'progress' with the democracy, good governance and efficiency (Apter, 1965). Inkleles (1974) from a socio- psychological point of view justified modernisation for an independent, rational and modern outlook. Consequently, as a process, modernisation is seen as means of social life or organization which emerged in Europe and became a worldwide phenomenon (Giddens, 1991).

Modernisation has also been distinguished by the notion of superiority of secular, materialistic and Western individualistic culture (Lerner, 1958; Schramm, 1964) dismissing cultural practices particularly faith and religion, as obstacles to progress (Bellah, 1965). The influence of Comte and Marxism led to the questioning of the role of faith, tradition and culture in the social life, which eventually meant a progressive rationalization and secularization of society and the dominance of science over traditional beliefs (Dallmayr, 1993). These arguments point towards similarities in the construction of the discourse of developmentalism in the 'Third World' and that of the social exclusion in the West, as both processes use modernisation as a conceptual tool for selection and rejection. While in the poor countries, the yardstick of modernity, progress and economic betterment is used to dismiss people's faith, tradition and cultural practices as the bottleneck to development, in the West similar tools are applied in othering and eventually marginalising people.

Modernisation theories generally seen to be the offshoot of the theories of social evolution which saw human societies seeking to increase their survival chances like the neo-Darwinian concepts of natural selection. Influenced by Spencer and Durkheim, modernisation theorists argued that societies and cultures develop over time like a living organism, making progress through several stages. At the macro level, the social evolution influenced the way development was conceived and practiced, leading to important concepts in sociology of development, especially bipolar theories of modernization, which in turn distinguished societies in terms of traditional versus modern.

Most communication practices and scholarship in the development literature reflect the overarching dominance of modernisation as the process and goal of social change. Three distinct phases of the role of communication, especially mass media in the process of development can be identified. In the first phase, after the World War II mass media was seen to support economic development through diffusion of technical and social innovations and prepare the human mind to change from a traditional to a modern outlook (McQuail, 2000). In the second phase which emerged from critical theory, modernisation was criticized as a Western cultural and economic imperialism or dominance (Schiller, 1976). The last phase has been mainly concerned about the contradictions in the modernisation process and the consequences of information and communication technologies on individuals in contemporary society (Giddens, 1991).

Many critical scholars, especially those from the 'Third World', ethnic, feminist and indigenous persuasions, supported by some Western scholars have criticized modernisation for its internal theoretical inconsistencies and its built-in asymmetry and political-economic inequity (Dallmayr, 1993). Majid Rahnema went further to argue that the scarcities attributed to the traditional societies were not due to the lack of their productive capacities, but to adherence to a completely different 'philosophy of being and relating with each other where people tried to make the 'best of what God or Nature had given them, than to divert all their energies to producing and making more money'. Highly critical of the modernisation process, Rahnema writes that the rationale of modernisation creates 'modernized poverty' which, he argues, incapacitates people by increasing the gap between the socially induced needs and their 'inability to meet those needs' (2001:3). In a detailed critique of modernisation, Tariq Banuri (1990) writes that the process of modernisation disenfranchises people and takes peoples' focus away from their own worldviews to the dominant worldview of the West:

> *...the project of modernisation has been deleterious to the welfare of 'Third World' population not because of bad policy advice or malicious intent of the advisers, nor because of the disregard of neo-classical wisdom, but rather because the project has constantly forced indigenous people to divert their energies from the positive pursuit of indigenously defined social change, to the negative goal of resisting cultural, political and economic domination of the West.* (1990:66)

The dominant paradigm of development was instrumental in the formulation of development communication theory and practice. Everett Rogers (1976: 121) observed, —this concept of development grew out of historical events such as Industrial Revolution in Europe and United States, the colonial experience in Latin America, Africa and Asia, the quantitative empiricism of North American social sciences, and capitalist economic/political philosophy. Obviously, anything traditional was seen as incompatible with modernity. Culture and faith were seen as impediments to change. Weber (1964), one of the proponents of modernity as a pre requisite for change, particularly, saw Oriental values and religions without a Protestant ethic to be a bottleneck to industrial capitalism (Singer, 1972).

These views render the non-Western world inferior and unfit for change. The Muslim world, in particular, is seen stagnant, and the practices, experiences and institutions of people living under varied social, cultural, political and economic conditions in this 'world are essentialised as a consequence of Islam itself and 'not as a result of specific political or socio–economic situations'. (Munoz, 2002, The Imperial Imagery. Para, 6). Against this backdrop, the stereotypical images of Muslim women are often used to endorse and project preconceived notions about Islam in the West. Munoz further writes:

> *By contrast, the values of the West are presented as a unique paradigm applicable to the whole of humanity, so that cultural diversity is experienced, not as a variety of options of equal value, but as a hierarchical structure in the scale modernisation backwardness. This ethnocentric cosmopolitanism, which exclusively attributes to itself the paradigm of rationality and progress, tends to define the Muslim world as remote from modernity.* (Ibid)

This process dialectically supports processes of modernisation by making words more important than objects. Many poststructuralism influenced scholars like Sachs (1990), Crush (1995) and Escobar (1992, 1995a, b) believe that it is this discourse of developmentalism that created the 'Third World' along with the processes and institutions to manage it. Steeve and Melkote (2001: 92), examining the modernisation discourse, argue that the goal from the beginning was to change the non-Western way of life with the Western one to 'reshape the reality of people in the Third World'. Consequently, the Western conception of progress and development took over the 'knowledge system' and 'existential reality' of the people.

In the context of the 'Third World', the experiential knowledge of people was made to follow the scientific pursuits, as their lives were considered to be laden with problems that could only be resolved by becoming modern. This also paved the way for agencies and institutions to intervene. Escobar (1992: 22) observes that this construction of social problems through the process of modernisation forced individuals to imagine their 'underdevelopment', and visualize there was something wrong with their way of life. Not far from this discursive practice, through the spatial reach of discursive power, the 'inner city' is constructed in the UK. Within this space, the bi-polar theories of modernisation are once again used. The traditional/modern debate is repeated through exclusion/inclusion. The inner city is the 'Third World' of the 'First world' and people who live in these spaces are reduced to problems that need to be solved. In the both the academic and policy debate, the inner city and marginalized existences are intertwined into labels like degeneration, deprivation, disadvantage and so on.

Although many disadvantaged people manage their lives and seek support from within the communities they live in, their ability and capacity to deal with exclusion on the basis of their experience and faith is not recognized. Pierson (2004: 191) argues that behind the numbers and figures which link people belonging to minority ethnic communities to exclusion, 'there are people with strengths, skills and resilience for dealing with adverse conditions'. These strengths often emerge from Biradaris,[2] religious affiliations and social relationships. During my observation, the author found some people living in Forest Fields, Hyson Green, Radford, Lenten and Sneinton in Nottingham relying on these communal networks for help and support. One popular way used by the members of the ethnic minority communities, especially by the Mirpuri and Bengali people, to help each other, is what is known locally as 'committee' – type of an informal and unregulated credit union. The members of the 'committee' make weekly contributions and help those people in financial difficulty. Although the beneficiary has to be a member, he/she gets a loan amount interest free without any paper work and guarantee. This way people who need startup capital for buying a taxi or starting small grocery or a 'take-away' are given a loan which they reimburse through small weekly installments. These 'committees' are run purely on trust and reciprocity which is more common among the closely knit communities. In most of the cases, such committees are operated by women who run small boutiques, tailoring or book shops in the area. This arrangement works well within minority groups, mostly concentrated in particular areas of the city where the mainstream banks and other financial institutions have limited presence. According to Kempson and Whyley (1999), some minority ethnic groups – 'particularly Pakistani and Bangladeshi households – make limited use of financial products due to language barriers, religious beliefs and lack of knowledge'. Within these circumstances the networks based on kinship and faith work well.

The research into the relationship between faith and development in the UK is sporadic, but more often it has been observed that within the marginalised communities, especially in the poorest neighbourhoods, religious group 'maintain some voice', providing an 'incredible source of energy' to empower people (Pierson, 2004: 184). The faith-based institutions, churches, mosques, gurdawaras and temples have become proactive in working with statutory organisations to address the issues of health inequalities. For example, smoking cessation campaigns like the QUIT and the 'New Leaf' have successfully worked with mosques in Nottingham to raise awareness about giving up smoking. Similarly, the vaccination against the spread of contagious diseases during the annual Hajj pilgrimage has become very successful in the UK by involving religious institutions and mosques in this process. Many mosques and community centres are now running healthy living centres for women and old people from minority ethnic groups to provide services within culturally sensitive environment. (For more details see, MCB and Muslim Health Networks websites)

Tariq Modood (1998), argues that ethno-religious groups, which are an important part of the minority identity and culture, are absent from social policy debate. He regrets an important source of 'renewal of community', which can provide 'compassion, fairness, justice and public morality' is hardly present in both the theory and practice of fighting social exclusion in the UK. Instead the numbers both at local and national level replace experience as institutions and processes are created to intervene, and progress is measured through quantitative number crunching. Within the dominant paradigm, mass media are generally attributed an uncritical role in development. Some communication and development scholars believed that an increased exposure to mass media, especially television, can increase the process of modernisation (Rogers, 1969; Lerner, 1958; Schramm, 1964). As this dominant paradigm started coming under the scrutiny of critical and liberatory perspectives, the power of mass media in transforming people from 'traditional to modern' was also questioned. Central to the scheme of modernisation has been the socio-scientific foundation of communication, which has over-emphasized the role of mass media through effects, modernisation and the diffusion of innovation approach along with social marketing. The current use of Information Communication Technology (ICT) also falls within this paradigm.

All these approaches have, in one way or another, paid no heed to the spatio-temporal realities in which people live. In other words, the context in which people live, their culture and tradition has been made redundant and irrelevant to the process of their development. Whether these communication models had Western bias, innovation bias, effects bias, source bias or increased the knowledge gap, these approaches did not bring any qualitative change in the lives of people (Bordenave & Diaz, 1977). Daniel Lerner (1958) argued that the social, economic and political development was proportional to the manifestation of mass media, implying that such media were the mediator as well as a yardstick for measuring the development.

By the 1970's it was becoming clear that the process of development was not straight forward, and in Latin America and Asia it was seen that social and economic constraints were too big and powerful to be changed by mass media (Rogers, 1976). Similarly, the diffusion of innovations approach, which used persuasion and technology to 'bring change', was criticized for its' 'pro innovation', 'pro-content' and one-way flow bias. It was found that this approach actually widens the information and material gaps among the farmers in the 'Third World'.

The diffusion of innovation practice was seen more of a quantitative approach that did not give qualitative insights into respondents (Golding, 1974). Other practices, like social marketing, and now the much-publicised use of Information Communication Technology (ICT) have not had much impact on development. While the former is seen a tool for the elite and government for 'social engineering', the impact of the latter is yet to be ascertained. There is a growing concern over the possibility of ICT leading to 'knowledge gap', as not many poor people have means and access to technology to use it to overcome the social, cultural and economic hurdles they face (Heeks, 1999:15). There are, however, some case studies in the 'Third World' were ICT is proving beneficial in rural development (Grameen Telecommunication Project in Bangladesh, National Association of Software Services Companies NASSCOM in Mumbai), but these are sporadic cases and the real benefit of such technology can only be assessed when people have universal access, skills and means to use technology. The decade of the 90's witnessed a major shift in traditional thinking about development and social change, bringingin the people-centred perspective, which took into cognizance the context in which development takes place. First there was debate on sustainable development, which brought issues of the environment following the Rio de Janeiro conference in 1992. Similarly respect for human life and concern for human rights was brought into the development debate following the Human Rights Conference in Vienna in 1993. After 1995 there was a renewed discussion on basic needs orientation, focusing on participatory approaches in communication and strengthening of critical consciousness and greater emphasis on community. This approach has led to the formulation of empowerment strategies. These debates took place at a time when postmodernism, post-structuralism and feminist scholarship challenged the logo- centric and ethno-centric views and models. Questions were asked about the universal truths and notions of objective social reality. Understanding diversity, dissension, and sensitivity towards ethnic issues became part of the wider debate. All this, finally brought the ethical dimension to the development discourse, stressing self-reliant, participatory and empowerment-related outcomes, in which tradition and culture are not seen as bottlenecks.

Although the dominant paradigm is said have passed, power relations within new models do not seem to be displaced as participation is often induced, directed, and co-opted. (Melkote & Steeves, 2001: 339). The bottom-up strategies have thus turned out to be clichés devoid of any substance. Despite the wide ranging critique of developmentalism emerging from the post colonial, post structural, feminist and other critical perspectives, the discourse of development, influenced mainly by the process of modernisation, continued to shape the national and international policies on change, progress and growth. Many substitutes, in the shape of anti-development, market-friendly development, autonomous development, sustainable development and so on, have failed to provide a model that can conceptualise development outside the 'normalised' discourse of development. For decades, development has remained confined within developmentalism.

Much of today's academic work in development support communication is premised on pluralistic and participatory approaches as opposed to the top to bottom perspective transmission models of the past but, even now, many of the frameworks offered today do not significantly differ from the dominant paradigm. The structure of elite domination has not changed. Bordenave (1980) noted that in these new approaches the sources and change agents often direct that participation. It is believed that marginalized people are often co-opted in activities whose results are pre-determined to increase agricultural production, improving education or increasing consumption.

There is a parallel between these approaches and the way the socially excluded are further marginalized by the media discourse in the West. Minorities, whether defined by language, religion, ethnicity, gender or sexual orientations, are pushed to the margins by the mainstream media. With corporate and state use of communication being seen further making media out of bounds for social gain (Wasko & Mosco, 1992), locally organised media are increasingly becoming the 'voice' of the voice-less. Many critical scholars have underlined the importance of small-scale media in alternative communication. Hollander and Stappers (1992) believe this type of communication serves as a frame of reference for shared interpretation of the topics communicated within the community.

As mentioned earlier in this chapter, this study, while using a number of perspectives to examine the social policy vis-à-vis fighting exclusion draws on the lessons learnt from a community radio station in Nottingham in contextualising people-centred efforts in this regard. Radio Ramzan caters to the community of South Asian immigrants, mostly from the Mirpuri district of the Pakistan Administered Kashmir, although there are other Muslims from Pakistan, India and Bangladesh and some from the Middle East living in Nottingham. The Mirpuri community has created its own spaces in the UK by living in clusters mostly in inner city areas. The Nottingham inner city has a significant presence of this community, which suffers from a wide range of social, economic, cultural and political problems.

Social Exclusion in the West

Despite unclear definitions, social exclusion dominates the social policy debate in the UK. The policy documents that determine government thinking show that explanation of social exclusion is ambiguous and imprecise (Byrne, 1999; Atkinson & Davoudi, 2000). This does not stop politicians and policy makers use and abuse the term. Its frequent use in social policy, academia, media and political rhetoric has created a discourse of social exclusion very similar to the discourse of developmentalism in the 'Third World', but whether the concept helps to explain deprivation and inequality is debatable. Power and Wilson (2000), however, find one common theme in various explanations of the term: Social exclusion is about the inability of our society to keep all groups and individuals within reach of what we expect as a society (2000: 1).

In the UK various government policies highlight the growing importance given to fighting social exclusion by promising to include all its citizens in the social and economic prosperity, and providing an equal opportunity to all (SEU, 2000, 2001). The term may be new to the UK but it has been in use in France for over three decades where it denoted 'people and places' that society had left behind 'and cut off' from the mainstream national life (Hardill et al., 2001). Others see it a 'deprivation that is primary economic' (Bowring, 2000) and some even suggest that focus on social exclusion means 'return to the politics of social justice' (Hague et al., 1999). With this vagueness, some say that social exclusion can cover anyone or anything (Saunders & Tsumori, 2002). Many scholars have warned about the fuzziness of the concept, and the carelessness about its use (Madanipour et al., 1998). Social scientists find the rhetorical use of social exclusion as a reason for giving it such a high profile within social policy especially since social exclusion was introduced in the European Community policy in 1980 (Berghman, 1997; Levitas, 1998; Marsh & Mullins, 1998). Levitas not only finds the definition of social exclusion problematic but also its measurement tricky:

> In an ideal world, definition precedes decisions about measurement, or where direct measurement is impossible, choice of proxy indicators. Part of the difficulty of finding indicators of social exclusion is that there is no agreed definition either of the phenomenon itself or of its main causes. (Levitas, 1999: 16)

Finding the current work on social exclusion inadequate and lacking clarity, Levitas argues that this inadequacy only helps politicians 'pick and mix' among indicators, and to justify preferred policies to avoid confronting the growth of poverty and income inequality. The conflicting explanations of social exclusion coming from a variety of disciplines and political persuasions make the concept very adaptable; consequently the concept is understood differently in different parts of the world. Silver (1994) classified social exclusion within national conceptions of what should keep society together. He advocated the solidarity perspective in France, depicting loss of social bonds, the spatalisation perspective in the US, denoting discrimination and segregation, and the monopoly perspective in the Western Europe, showing exclusion as a result of group domination. This classification points to the multi-dimensional conceptualisation of the term, which many scholars find close to notions of social integration in different parts of the world.

At the same time, the fluidity of the concept and its multi-dimensional use is seen to be useful in explaining the diversity of causes and consequences of social exclusion (Madanipour et al., 1998). These scholars emphasise the concepts usefulness in highlighting everyday life situations where inequalities arise. They also emphasise the importance of making links across these dimensions. Whatever the precise definition, social exclusion in the UK is thought to be a result of the fall-out from the globalisation of labour, production and finance. Evidence indicates that the 'Thatcher project' has helped particular sections of British society to gain financially. Globalisation, which gained currency in the early nineties, further facilitated this gain for the few at the expense of the majority of the poor. While the privileged are benefiting, the less privileged are being excluded, living marginal lives away from the glamour of the new economic reality. Many among the underprivileged are people belonging to ethnic minorities. The decline of the manufacturing industry, where most of the South Asian first generation migrants worked, forced them into a spiral of poverty and deprivation.

But how do the policy makers define social exclusion? The Social Exclusion Unit (SEU) in its report, 'Minority ethnic issues in social exclusion and neighbourhood renewal (2000) says that social exclusion includes 'poverty and low income', but is broader and addresses some of the wider causes and consequences of poverty. The unit defines social exclusion as:

> *a shorthand term for what can happen when people or areas suffer from a combination of linked problems such as unemployment, poor skills, low incomes, poor housing, high crime, bad health and family breakdown.* (SEU, 2000)

The government strategy has come under heavy criticism from various quarters. First and foremost, the policy sees an economic rationale in including those excluded. This approach does not look at non-material aspects of life and experience. Scholars dismiss the number-crunching explanation of exclusion and argue for a wider concept that looks at the context of social exclusion. In her pioneering discourse analysis, Levitas (1999) argues that there are at least three ways of looking at the issue:

> *Moral Underclass Discourse* (MUD), which puts blame for exclusion on those being excluded by playing down the inequalities inherent in society. Within this discourse, those seeking state help are demonised as an 'underclass'. *Social Integrationist Discourse* (SID) where the route to inclusion is through paid work and those not in jobs are seen having 'no morals'. *Radical Egalitarian Discourse* (RED): Here the structural inequalities as a result of market capitalism lead to proposals for a redistribution agenda for change. Levitas thinks that the Labour government's social policy revolves around these three discourses. However, there seems to be a transition from a RED perspective to the SID perspective, which is increasingly becoming part of the European policy as well (1999: 22). Levitas sees a pattern in the shift of focus to SID and MUD from RED as New Labours' attempt to de-link social exclusion from poverty and justify actions that do not necessarily address the issues of redistribution of material goods. There is also a contrast between the political rhetoric and actual policy, which can be gauged from this transition. The Labour government's approach in dealing with social exclusion is also believed to take a simplistic view of those being

excluded by ignoring the cultural diversity and social complexity which defines contemporary inner city areas.

Another feature of social exclusion discourse is its conceptual softness, which New Labour exploits to use to show off in dealing with some of the very high profile social issues. Burchardt et al. (2002) argue that policy makers have concentrated on the most visible and extreme issues which are likely to capture the attention of the wider public, such as street homelessness, teenage mothers, drug related crime, and policies to reduce anti-social behaviour. The structural flaws are also blamed for the failures in the past to promote inclusion and equality along with lack of consistent national approach, which implies that services have often worked in parallel, not in a 'joined-up' way (Social Exclusion Unit, 2000). So, the 'joined-up' services and organisations, agencies and local businesses working in partnership, became the new buzzword in the development of the government's social policies. But this mantra has been criticised for creating mega bureaucracies to deal with the localised complex social issues. Levitas (1999) and Bowring (2000), argue that the emphasis on joined up government makes accountability harder to enforce, as it is difficult to trace specific policies and their effects.

The government department responsible for fighting social exclusion accepts the deficiency in recognizing this complexity. The socially excluded people are disproportionately concentrated in deprived areas and suffer all the problems that affect other people in these areas, but people from minority ethnic communities also suffer the consequences of:

> *Overt and inadvertent racial discrimination – individual and institutional, an inadequate recognition and understanding of the complexities of minority ethnic groups, and hence services that fail to reach them or meet their needs; and additional barriers like language, cultural and religious differences but in practice very little is done to address the problem.* (SEU, 2000)

One set of reasons cannot hold good for every individual and group. This implies a relational understanding of the concept in which presence/absence of links connections and networks play a greater role in explaining exclusion than structural processes that were believed to be responsible for inequality. Room (1995) thinks that social exclusion can be better understood by putting greater emphasis on relational processes that keep people away from participating in social and economic activities. However, the connection between relational factors and material deprivation is not a new concept. Townsend (1979:31) writes that poverty is a process where people are 'being excluded from ordinary living patterns customs and activities'. This definition is not very different from present discourse on social exclusion. But what is new is the way the agency and capacity in combating social exclusion have been appropriated into this discourse.

Creation of managerial strategies to deal with 'social disorder' is not a new thing. Cowen and Shenton (1995) observe that idea of development was in vogue in Europe in the nineteenth century as it was used to sort out social chaos caused as a result of poverty, unemployment and rapid urbanization. The riots in Burnley, Bradford and other northern towns of England echoed this chaos in the summer of

2001. These riots revealed the extent of social division on one hand and on the other showed levels of deprivation experienced by the people living in these areas (Cantle report, 2001). These disturbances, which shook the foundations of multiculturalism and the notion of equality in the UK, took place despite the government's claims to be spending millions to address the issues of perennial disaffection experienced by people living in the run-down city areas.

The then Home Secretary established a review team, led by Ted Cantle, to seek the views of local residents and community leaders in the affected towns and in other parts of England in order to bring about social cohesion and also to identify good practice in the handling of these issues at the local level. The Cantle report, which was published in December 2001, revealed the physical segregation of housing estates and inner city areas and the depth of polarisation in British towns and cities. The report coined the famous phrase 'parallel lives' to focus on the physical divisions between communities compounded by separate educational arrangements, community and voluntary bodies, employment, places of worship, language, social and cultural networks.

The report remarked that the whole 'equalities' agenda has become heavily associated with black and ethnic minority groups despite efforts to promote a more inclusive agenda (2001:10). This report suggested that such approach leads to an assumption that 'black and ethnic minority groups are in need, and that they are seen as recipients'. Although the Cantle report mostly looked at the consequences of this segregation, at some places it revealed the extent of disadvantage faced by the people belonging to minority ethnic groups:

> *We recognised that some communities felt particularly disadvantaged and that the lack of hope and the frustration borne out of poverty and deprivation all around them meant that disaffection would grow. Yet they were not always well targeted, nor even identified. For example, some black and ethnic minorities felt that they were always identified without sufficient differentiation and 'problematised' as a result. Similarly, some poorer white communities also felt left out completely like the members of the black and minority ethnic groups.* (Cantle, 2001: 11)

Racism in the form of Islamophobia was also identified as a problem in the areas, and for 'some young people was part of their daily experience'. The report suggested that these young people felt that there were 'being socially excluded because of their faith'. While problematising communities are part of the discourse that creates inner city ghettoes, efforts to address the issues of poverty and discrimination were seen to 'institutionalise the problems'. The plethora of initiatives and programmes, with their baffling array of outcomes, boundaries, timescales and other conditions, seemed to ensure divisiveness and a perception of unfairness in virtually every section of the communities we visited...The most consistent and vocal concern was expressed about the damaging impact of different communities bidding against each other and the difficulty of being able to convince them about the fairness of the present approach...Reference was constantly made to the fact that new initiatives are constantly being introduced, even before old ones have been completed; that national schemes, with national derived targets and priorities, disempower local communities; and that the complexity of bidding and funding arrangements take up disproportionate amounts of time (2001: 25)

The Cantle report did not specifically look at the role of media in the riots, but recorded complaints about the local media for its bias and misrepresentation. A number of respondents blamed the press and media for stirring up racial tension in order to titillate readers and sell more papers. They called for measures to make the press and media more accountable and responsible. The importance of local press and media was also emphasised. In the recent disturbances, it was suggested that a number of local editors were particularly irresponsible in their selection of letters for publication (2001:64)

The inquiry into the causes and consequences of these riots has demonstrated that assimilation and integration models have not worked. Consequently, the model of social cohesion based on the 'European Social Model' which acknowledges the existence of disparities within and between groups was suggested. This model emphasizing 'mutual support' and 'shared social goals', nonetheless faces a number of questions. With the debate on immigration and multiculturalism becoming one of the major political issues in the Europe, minority groups are demanding social justice as 'different equals'. Against this background, the Cantle report has been criticised for its 'insensitivity' towards the difference and has been lamented for putting the blame for deprivation on the victims of deprivation. The report has focused attention on social isolation, which is an outcome of the exclusion. There are push factors like racism, lack of culturally sensitive provisions and facilities, and there are some pull factors like, strong family connections, cultural practices and lack of exposure responsible for this phenomenon. Discrimination, both at individual and institutional level, is recognised as one of the main reasons for social exclusion, but it is also the lack of voice, stereotyping which force people to look inwards for help and support.

The literature explains how symbolic boundaries arise between racially constructed categories (Hall, 1992a, b:255) and how these representations are generalized, perpetuated and legitimised through the media and official discourses. The differences of religion, custom and cultures among the racially constructed groups are exploited by the media, which leads to hostility and suspicion between the groups. A close examination of the situation reveals that official, political and media discourses work hand in hand to demonise difference for their individual and sometimes mutual interest. Calling the process of managing people's lives a discourse of 'governmentality', Clarke (2000: 110) from a Foucauldian analysis, argue that activation, empowerment, responsibilization and abandonment constitute four dynamics of the process of governmentality, of which New Labour appear as exemplary practitioner. Through this process, Clarke (Ibid) write that citizens are transformed into subjects who understand themselves as responsible and independent agents.

These scholars find the 'revelatory style' of Foucauldian analysis helpful in uncovering the complex and subtle workings of power. Production of self- regulating subjects as job seekers, marginalised, inner city dwellers, illegal immigrants, hardworking families, socially excluded, and so on, are categories used to manage diversity. Such an approach not only serves as a convenient means of categorisation which essentialises difference but is also used as a pretext to pass the blame of exclusion, underachievement in education, higher unemployment and poor health to the victims of inequality. The official discourse for its own bureaucratic and administrative convenience uses categories like 'disaffected', 'disenfranchised', 'low achievers', 'low skilled', 'less healthy', 'discriminated' and so on to refer to people and spaces which exist outside the 'normal' West. These categories enter into political discourse where terminology changes but meanings remain the same.

The symbols become very important, as 'immigrant', 'refugees', 'asylum seekers, 'ethnic minorities', 'non-white', 'coloured', 'black', 'faith based' are used indiscriminately by politicians to grab headlines and catch the attention of the voters. And the media, especially the tabloid press, further sensationalise the difference by demonising the 'other'. So the headlines like 'swamping of our schools and hospitals', 'Terrorists in the neighbourhood', 'Parallel Lives' and 'Forced marriages; enter into the public domain. The media in the UK has used immigration and asylum on many occasions to do scaremongering, and politicians use these headlines to score points. The issue has got so muddled up that it is very difficult to make a distinction between a foreign worker, an immigrant, a refugee, an asylum seeker and so on. Immigration in itself has emerged as a serious discourse in European politics in the Post War era, and in the UK this discourse has taken centre stage in defining national and local policies vis-à-vis this discourse. Many studies and reports into the issues of social exclusion have indicated this relationship as the proportion of minority ethnic groups mostly belonging to the generation of immigrant communities are disproportionately caught in the cycles of unemployment, poor health, poor housing, low educational achievement and higher incidents of racism and higher dependence on benefits (MacPherson Report, 1999; Cantle Report, 2001) street. In Nottingham, for example, the majority of the Muslim community is living in the Hyson Green, Lenton and Sneinton areas of the city. These areas with established facilities like mosques, specialised groceries, take-aways, cloth – shops and charities, have for long provided people a network and support to live together. A similar pattern can be seen in all major towns of the UK where minorities, especially Pakistani/ Mirpuri can be seen living together. In fact, the largest population of Mirpuris outside the Mirpur in Pakistan Administered Kashmir is believed to be in Birmingham (150,000). Various explanations have been given for this phenomenon including the support network, fear of racism, convenience etc. (Lewis, 1994).

But these spaces have become the focus of many studies, as these areas reveal notable deprivation, and people living in these areas are disadvantaged in many ways. There is a sense of rejection and exclusion among the people from the mainstream, but at the same time there is a strong desire to live together as a community, though a multiplicity of ambiguities and differences exists between and within the groups of people. The idea of the community provides a refuge from the hostile environment and a platform to contest these hostilities. Jeffery (1976:182) highlights this pull factor by referring to studies that suggest and support the idea that 'conscious re-assertion of Pakistani-ness is a probable response to such rejection' by the indigenous population. Whether inspirational or real, the idea of communal living gives rise to particularities, which are used to assert the identity. Raghuram sees this revival of religion as an expression of socio-cultural particularism against the universalizing tendencies of globalisation, though she thinks this distinction is unstable (Raghuram, 1999).

Most of the work carried out on the theme of faith and regeneration explores the role faith communities play in urban development. Farnell writes that the majority of the research undertaken in this area involves the faith communities themselves, usually in an attempt to evaluate the effectiveness of current activity. In the early 1990's a study of the community impact of the Church Urban Fund was published, funded in part by the central government. 'Hope in the City' drew conclusions about the Fund's impact in Manchester, Birmingham and Southwark (Farnell et al., 1994). Recommendations were made which have subsequently influenced an agenda for the fund's development.

Papers stemming from this work were published in community empowerment, community organizing and community initiatives in relation to state urban policy. 'Faith in the city' and the Church Urban Fund have been the focus of a number of higher degree dissertation on Church engagement in community development. However, it is argued that regeneration is a signifier of profound change in many religious traditions and political ideologies, both radical and conservative (Furbey 1999). According to Musgrave (1998), only a few community based initiative within News deal for communities project have shown the positive outcomes faith can play in neighbourhood renewal.

Taking account of the role faith can play in regeneration; the government has included in its policy the input from the Inner City Religious Council (ICRC) to make a lasting impact on the lives of people who live in these areas. Since its creation in 1992 the Inner City Religious Council (ICRC), has included representatives of five of the largest faith communities in England: Christians, Hindus, Jews, Muslims and Sikhs. It is chaired by a government minister and provides a forum where they and the government can work together on urban renewal and social inclusion. The ICRC is part of the Urban Policy Unit – formed to take forward the agenda of the Urban White Paper published in November 2000. But the role of the ICRC is only consultative, while the actual implementation of projects is carried out with tested and trusted means and practices, where numbers and not experiences are counted.

In fact, the New Labour government was criticised for being too managerial in its approach in dealing with perennial social problems. The emergence of the 'managerial state', a businesslike organising, which counts efficiency through setting of targets and hiring of more managers (Clarke, 2000), is believed to ignore the holistic, contextual approach. This approach can be best demonstrated the way New Labour has been managing the National Health Service (NHS).

Faith, Place and Exclusion

Traditionally, the process of development based on the Western worldview, sees religion and other forms of faith in conflict with 'progress and change'. Literature within this discourse suggests that non-material variables only become important when they are perceived as problems and 'stigmatized as inferior in culture, religion or race' (Friberg & Hettene, 1985). Non-Western faiths like Islam, Buddhism and Hinduism are especially seen to create barriers for progress (Melkote & Steeves, 2001). But with the growing criticism of the developmentalism, coinciding with the growth in alternative movements, there is a heightened consciousness about the importance of religion and culture in contextualizing development as a people- centred endeavour (Wang & Dissanayake, 1984; Servaes, 1999). Within the cultural practice of the marginalized communities, identity as a worldview shaped by unique epistemology, historiography and philosophy of life is seen by many scholars to play a significant role in the re-conceptualisation of development to displace the Western world-view. Sardar, indicating the 'power shift towards non-Western ways of doing things', argues that 'there will be more than one dominant way of being human, of being free, and there will be more than one way to develop' (Sardar, 1997: 47).

Liberation theology, which evolved from Latin America, supports development as a 'process of personal and communal liberation', where 'empowerment and self-reliance' should be the goal of such development. It suggests emancipatory communication, where interpersonal and group strategies lead to 'expanded consciousness' consistent with the 'spiritual practice' and faith of people. Under this perspective power shifts from external factors to 'individuals, organizations, and communities over social and economic conditions, over political processes and over their own stories' (Melkote & Steeves, 2001: 366). However, the relationship between religion and development is not well researched. Exploring this area (Raghuram, 1999), writes that literature on the relationship between religion and development is patchy, although 'economic development is often viewed as being essentially secular' (Raghuram, 1999: 238).

Exploring the implicit and explicit ways in which religion and development contest, Raghuram (ibid) concludes that 'religion and development are interlinking processes, which engage with each other to produce change'. Citing the example of emphasis in the Protestant tradition on individualism, she explains how this reformist movement promoted capitalist economic development. At the same time, she writes about the static nature of other faiths like Islam and Confucianism to impede development. Thus, she remarks that religion can be a seedbed for development while development can instigate religious change. The static/dynamic nature of faiths is debatable. Religions in pure form have brought sea changes. Whether the Hinduism-inspired Sarvodhya movement in India or the Islamic concept of Zakat (obligatory charity) or Protestant inspired Capitalism, faiths have changed the course of the world and continue to influence and shape the spiritual, social, cultural and political life of millions of people. However, in many parts of the world, religions have adapted to local social and cultural situations, and the 'stagnation', which the religion has widely been accused of, could be part of that local variation or misinterpretation of the religions. Islam, for example, puts explicit emphasis on change and seeking change: —Allah does not change the condition of any nation unless it strives in that direction (Qur'an, 13/11: 8/53). Ilm (Knowledge) is the seed-bed for such a change. Allah is Aleem (most knowledgeable) and seeking knowledge is made mandatory for both men and women. Prophet Muhammad (PBUH5) reinforced this message by saying in of his Hadith that knowledge should be sought even if one has to go to China. This stress on seeking knowledge is not just the revealed but also the acquired knowledge, which Choudury (1992: 60) describes as 'an evolutionary process embracing interactive intelligence and experience gained in all sub-systems of the universe'.

Historically, Islam in its simple message has been committed to the liberation of the poor and encouraging pluralism. From the early days of Islam when Prophet Muhammad (PBUH) was establishing the first community of Muslims in Medina, the inner dynamism of Islam started unfolding. This theology of liberation was actually put in practice by Prophet Muhammad (PBUH) when he, through his own word and action, challenged ignorance, oppression and injustice. Asghar Ali Engineer, a renowned scholar from the Indian subcontinent argues that such dignified ideals not only inspire and encourage, but also lead to purposeful action:

> *Also, Muhammad worked for the liberation of the oppressed, the poor and the needy and the ignorant. He was, in this project of liberation, not only a teacher and philosopher, but also an activist, participant and fighter. Under his inspiration, the Arabs not only liberated themselves but also sought to liberate others by shattering the two greatest oppressive empires of the world then i.e. the Roman and thee Sassanid. Their stormy victories were ensured, as they were seen by the oppressed of these mighty empires as liberators.* (Engineer, 2000)

The empowerment led liberation perspective, which 'prioritizes personal and communal liberation from oppression', is seen to make faith central to self- reliance and human emancipation. The concept of development as liberation as propagated by the Brazilian educator Paolo Freire (1972) is influenced by the Christian Liberation Theology6 which Gustavo Gutierrez, a Peruvian priest and theologian describes as being active on behalf of the poor, studying the Bible and praying. Steeve and Melkote (2001), quoting Gutierrez, believe that the liberation theology is based on the following tenets:

- *That God is very close to humanity,*
- *That we encounter God via commitment to justice to all,*
- *That a spirituality of liberation is inseparable from the work of liberation. (2001: 277–278)*

These tenets of Christian theology resonate in all major religions. Islam in particular, being an Ibrahim religion, has a similar set of guidelines regarding care, equality and social action.

The concept of liberation within Islamic literature is not well researched, though many Muslim and non-Muslim scholars would argue that whole philosophy of

Islam is based on human liberation, dignity and justice (Smith, 1959; Esak, 1997; Engineer, 2000). Commentators like Merryl Wyn Davies (2002), have even gone to the extent to argue that Europe has learnt the art of reasoning from Islam. Davies (2002) argues that 'Islam taught Europe the very idea of reason as well as how to reason' (Shared Cultures section, Para. 2)

Wilfred Cantwell Smith's knowledge of the Orient helped him not only to do research in primary sources of Islam, but also enabled him to have first-hand interaction with Islamic 'ulama' (scholars). Smith's (1959) work in understanding Islam's role, particularly in socio-spiritual development, led him to criticise the Christian association with the presumed political and technological superiority of the West. Having studied a wide range of Muslim communities in the Arab world, Turkey, Pakistan, India, and Indonesia, Smith commented that the 'religion is alive and dynamic' (1959: 297). Although a Christian missionary and seen by many in the Muslim world as an Orientalist, Smith's contribution to the liberatory aspects of Islam is believed to be convincing.

However, it was Farid Esak (1997) who put forward Quranic tenets of Islamic liberation theology, though this hermeneutics of liberation is in the context of South Africa. He writes:

- *Allah is constantly involved in the affairs of humankind,*
- *Allah is concerned with justice for oppressed,*
- *A full understanding of the Quran support for the oppressed requires*
- *full commitment to and engagement in the struggle for liberation.*

But the liberation standpoint within Islamic thought has been criticised by traditionalists who see it as a philosophy to appropriate religion to fit liberal paradigms. It is argued that Esack's conceptualisation of Islamic liberation theology is driven by praxis and not an abstract encounter with God and revelation. Murad (1998), as one of the vociferous critics of Esack, argues that Esack is following the footsteps of another modernist, Ameer Ali, 'who nearly a century ago re-examined the Qur'an to discover in its pages the entire moral code of Victorian England; (1998. Para, 2). Esack who is thought to have borrowed the ideas from the liberation theology of Gutierrez, was very active against apartheid in South Africa, and this association has become the focus of criticism for 'his admirable willingness to cooperate with Christian opponents of apartheid' (Murad, Ibid., Para9).

From a puritan point of view, encounters with God, revelations and the life (Sunnah and Hadith) of Prophet (PBUH) are not only indispensable part of one's faith, but also the guiding principles for dealing with the material world. Within this view, Esack's humanistic approach in dealing with inequality, oppression and discrimination is bound to invite criticism, especially from those who subscribe to the Saudi sponsored Wahabi and Salafi schools of thought. But Esack himself is not deviating from the basic principles of Islam. It is the way he interprets the verses of Quran and quotes the Hadith and Sunnah to relate religion to the contemporary social issues. Another issue that has generated criticism of Farid Esack's conceptualization of liberation theology is the way his ideas have been labeled and made to look divorced from the basic tenets of Islam. Many Western scholars and media have called his work as 'progressive' which is seen by many dovetailing with liberal values (Murad, Ibid). Islam, in theory, is considered to be a practical religion with no boundaries between the political, social and the spiritual aspects of life, but in practice, the social realities of many of its followers are distantfrom their spiritual experiences.

After 9/11, there has been a surge in the debate about the political aspects of Islam, especially the relation between Islam and the West, but the debates about the democracy, equality and social justice within Muslim societies have not picked up. Although Islam itself is not responsible for this social inertia, it is used by many to stifle the debate. Many scholars (Ishaq, 1997; Sardar, 2002; Engineer, 2007) are calling for Ijtihad[3] to narrow the gap between the social and spiritual in Islam. Esack's work, though controversial, is the beginning of this process where religion and liberation are not seen in conflict but complimenting to create a humane, just and equal society. Looking at the growth of Islam and its capacity to bring various tribes, factions, ethnicities and nationalities together indicates the humanistic values of this religion. Islam's power to galvanise movements against tyrannies and injustices show its innate nature to support the oppressed. It has appealed to a variety of people in various situations and has provided the spiritual and political stimulation for many contemporary social and political movements in the world.

Malcolm X in the 1960's, preached and practicised a form of Islamic liberation theology during the Civil Rights Movement in the USA, which attracted millions of Black Americans. Similarly, Farid Esack propagated the Quranic hermeneutic of liberation in the context of the struggle against Apartheid in South Africa. The Iranian revolution, which ousted the autocratic Shah, led to a resurgence of Islamic movements against oppressive regimes in many other parts of the world. But at the same time, some extremist political and religious movements like the Taliban claim to be an Islamic movement, using Islam to promote its version of social justice. The Taliban phenomenon, which started as a student movement against the Soviet occupation of Afghanistan in due course of time became one of the most radicalized Islamic movements. Melkote and Steeves (2001) argue that as the Bible was used historically, some Muslim groups use the Quran in the same way to justify oppression and violence to suit their own narrow vision. However, the authors believe that the majority of Muslim opinion is against this fanaticism and has a more moderate outlook which is not represented in the contemporary media discourse, which they see as responsible for creating a non- representative image of Islam in the Western world. While the media are largely seen to be responsible for promoting negative images of Islam and Muslims, many Muslim scholars blame the oppressive regimes and despotic rulers for exploiting Islam for political reasons on the one hand, and the fanatic-preachers who use their literal, and what are seen by many as out of context, interpretations of Islam to legitimize their authority (Karawan, 1992; Sardar, 2002)

Ishaq Khan thinks the malaise in Muslim societies is a result of the influence of the Western ideologies:

... Rationalism, secularism, socialism, nationalism, liberalism and fundamentalism -or in other words, various forms of Western dogmatism – are more than mere forms of man's reason to reason out problems in the realm of mind Vis-a Vis society. Although, the Western society has not been monolithic in a strict sense, yet in one respect it has shown remarkable unity of purpose in its efforts in westernising the world in the name of ideologies. The West's worldview is, therefore, worldviews in a circumscribed sense. (Khan, 1997: 12)

The arguments between various shades of reformists, modernists, traditionalists and puritans are not new. Like many other contemporary Muslim scholars, Zia Uddin Sardar (2002) thinks that Muslims are caught in a struggle between the forces of 'secular modernity' fueled by globalization and a reactionary 'aggressive traditionalism'.

Sardar in his editorial comment, 'Islam: resistance and reform' (2002) puts the blame for this malaise on the 'history, social practice and intellectual and political inertia of Muslims themselves'. He argues that Muslims are not willing to reflect on the process. He believes that Muslims, on the whole, are very reluctant to look at themselves or to examine the processes that have 'transformed Islam into a suffocating and oppressive ideology'. Besides the lack of self-introspection, he thinks many Muslim societies have become authoritarian and despotic due to closing down of the possibility of Ijtihad, and non-adherence to the principles and practices adopted by Prophet Muhammad (PBUH). He argues:

Consider how the idea of ijma, the central notion of communal life in Islam, has been reduced to the consensus of a select few. Ijma literally means consensus of the people. The concept dates back to the practice of Prophet Muhammad himself as leader of the original polity of Muslims. When the Prophet Muhammad wanted to reach a decision, he would call the whole Muslim community – then admittedly not very large – to the mosque. A discussion would ensue; arguments for and against would be presented. Finally, the entire gathering would reach a consensus. Thus, a democratic spirit was central to communal and political life in early Islam. But over time the clerics and religious scholars have removed the people from the equation – and reduced ijma to 'the consensus of the religious scholars'. Not surprisingly, authoritarianism, theocracy and despotism reigns supreme in the Muslim world. (Sardar, 2002, p. 345)

This despondency, however, should not be associated with Islam itself. Engineer (2007) citing particular verses, argues that Quran clearly supports democratic Institutions as there are references in this holy book that Prophet Muhammad (PBUH) should consult his companions in all secular matters (3:158) and all Muslims should consult each other in their affairs (42:38). Islam as one of the largest faiths in the world is practiced by people of different colours, backgrounds and traditions in different parts of the world. Some of these countries are democratic, some autocratic while some are dictatorial, and in every setting the politicians, rulers and dictators use this religion for their own legitimacy. However, the social and political traditions of these countries and cultures are not necessarily Islamic but are pertinent to the region. There are many non-democratic Muslim countries where political institutions and democratic practices have not taken roots, but it is not because of Islam but due to the feudal structures and the tribal arrangements operational in these societies. In many Muslim countries, owing to their colonial past, dictatorships and monarchies have been traditionally supported by the Western countries, which have hampered the democratic process in these parts of the world.

However, in practice, Muslim world, as it exists today, is fragmented into sects and classes and many followers of the faith believe in their castes, clans and groups, which is a challenge to the universal concept of 'Ummah'. This fragmentation is further aggravated by the ongoing tussle between the modernist and traditionalist interpretations. Within Western scholarship, there are some scholars who see fundamentalism part of modernisation. Turner (2003) suggests that fundamentalism is a form of modernisation. Exploring the Nietzschean, Parsonian and McLuhanian paradoxes about the place of religion in the global age, he argues that the reformist philosophy of Islam supported the rational civilization, modern capitalism and democracy. He adds that the 'correct interpretation' of the Quran shows that Islam is compatible with modern science and rational thought (2003: 407). Bryan blames the pre-Islamic practices for the corruption, which he thinks comes in between Islam and modernity, and believes that 'fundamentalism is a solution for this corruption as it is a step towards modernisation' (Turner, 2003: 414).

However, many scholars see Muslim revival movements more as a reaction to the modernisation project of 'plutocracies' (Sayyid, 1997). What is being labelled as fundamentalism is seen by critical scholars as resistance to the universalisation of the Western knowledge as the only knowledge. Bobby Sayyid argues that through the orchestration of the 'Islamic way, Muslims voice an alternate subjectivity' in which Muslim identity encompasses all other identities, and where the 'language of Islamic metaphor is used to seek political destinies in a fragmented world' (1997:157).

Although Sayyid's (1997:73–74) analysis is more at a macro level, revealing many dimensions of the Islamic perspective vis-à-vis the West's modernisation project using Kemal Atta Turk's Turkey (Kemalist) and Khomeni's Iran as examples, this analysis is very relevant at a micro level when one explores the tensions and differences in the backyards of the West where a growing Muslim community is trying to define its existence on its own terms. Many second and third generation Muslims born and brought up in the UK foreground the Muslim identity in their political practice to demand state-funded Islamic schools, Muslim chaplaincy, Halal meals, Muslim media etc. Sayyid cites many reasons, including the domination of secular elites, the authoritarian nature of post-colonial regimes, uneven economic development, etc for the emergence of Islamism. The common denominator for colonization, secularization and developmentalism is seen to be the continuity of the 'West' as the only knowledge. The limit of Europe comes when groups of people begin to articulate their position on the basis of the rejection of Europe's claims to copyright (Sayyid, 1997: 17).

But the process of modernisation is not only criticized from the Islamic point of view. Many contemporary critical and emancipatory perspectives which argue for validation of other knowledges see modernisation as being racist, sexist and ignorant. Instead, faith, gender, ethnicity, sexualities and difference are seen as valid levels of analysis in exploring diversity of knowledge and the way (s) of living outside the notion of 'the knowledge' within the alternative scholarship (Melkote & Steeves, 2001). The pedagogic turn in development studies, often referred to as post development, is seen as very controversial by some academics who ridicule its simplistic explanations and 'lack of scholarship' (Corbridge, 1998). But this body of scholarship, nevertheless, has opened up the development discourse to a new level of analysis, which offers a variety of possibilities and potentialities of understanding why the development process has failed to engage with the people it was supposed to help.

With a renewed assertiveness among the minority ethnic groups, especially within the Muslim communities in UK gaining momentum, so is the desire among these groups to develop strategies and actions based on their experience and knowledge. Many such grassroots level social action programmes have become the focus of academic investigation. Many religious institutions including mosques are more proactive now to develop programs and strategies to help local people to improve health, education and employment in inner city areas. The Muslim Council of Britain (MBC) is currently involved in building the capacity of smaller community groups and mosques to access various streams of local, national and European funding for community development and fighting exclusion (MBC Website).

Although the role faith and cultural practices can play in helping people fight exclusion is not well researched, anecdotal evidence from poor parts of the world shows that the development strategies used within the context of faith have proved successful by increasing the participation of people and bringing qualitative changes in the lives of people (Esack, 1997). In the UK, political mobilization of ethnic minorities has largely remained confined around race relations. This mobilization, promoted on the principle of racial equality, has come under criticism for failing to understand the complexity of race and ignoring the spatio-temporal realities in which marginalized groups live. Difference, religion and ethnic origin have become the important areas of contestation and consensus within minorities. The focus is now shifting from a more generalised ethnic identity to a more specific religious identity.

The demands for equality and opportunity are not just made within broader racial categories, but within religious orientation, ethnic origin and nationality as well (Paul Statham, 1999). Tariq Modood, acknowledging the importance of religion in contemporary multicultural Britain, says that religious assertiveness among the South Asians is giving Britishness a new significance 'out of step with native trends', which he finds diversifying rather than segregating (Modood, 2004, TES). However, the conceptualization of faith-based interventions is meaningless unless such efforts take into consideration other critical perspectives that have, for different reasons and through different analyses, questioned the modernisation- inspired project of development. The critical scholarship may not agree on everything with the liberation perspectives, but all these standpoints seek pluralistic and egalitarian practices for the restoration of people's knowledge and capacity.

Although it is beyond the scope of this work to compare and contrast critical and liberatory standpoints, it is crucial to explore the common ground between these theories where emancipatory outcomes of my study can be grounded. Conceptualising such multi-perspective and multi-disciplinary framework is in conformity with the broader political agenda of this study.

Notes

1. MCB represents the interest of various Muslim organizations in the UK. It was founded in 1997. www.mcb.org.uk
2. Literally translated, Biradari means Kinship but in the Mirpuri politics it denotes the clan system- a social hierarchy that classifies people by their family professions.
3. The independent interpretation of problems/issues, not precisely covered by the Qur'an, Hadith and scholars. In the early Muslim community, adequately qualified jurist had the right to exercise such original thinking based on personal judgment and analogical reasoning. It was abandoned from the twelfth century when it was argued that Ijtihad can lead to errors and misinterpretation. The debate about Itihad has resurfaced as many Muslims struggle in resolving contemporary issues. There is a no consensus on the qualifications of a Mujtahid (one who can do Ijtihad).

Chapter 3
Epistemological Plurality

The preceding discussions in Chap. 2 highlighted the fact that the process of exclusion and marginalisation is a complex discourse of overlapping power relations, politics and subjectivities. This complexity cannot be explained and understood through a static mono-theoretical framework but will require a dynamic multi-disciplinary and multi-perspective methodology. Exploring exclusion, voice and agency, demands a strategic intersection of emancipatory, critical and spiritual perspectives to provide a non-essentialist outline to analyse the power relations and structures responsible for marginalisation on the one hand, and on the other offers ways of fighting back for the validation of the marginalised knowledge.

However, bringing faith, feminism and philosophy together is an audacious task. Allegiance to any one of these concepts can inhibit commitment to others (Groenhout, 2002). Philosophy is generally seen to be contrary to religious faith while the faith itself is believed to be averse to feminism. And feminism, by and large, has been against the male dominated philosophy. So where is a meeting point for these seemingly divergent concepts? Groenhout (Ibid), engaging with this difficult task, says that there is no single answer to how these, apparently differing, strands may come together, but she sees the range of approaches in addressing this dilemma leading to a framework which can, on the one hand, recognise the 'creative potential the tension between these allegiances may generate' and on the other, acknowledge the potential for 'creating mutually supportive coherence' out of these loyalties' (2002:11).

The conceptual, positional and methodological 'superiority' of Western knowledge has been contested from a variety of critical, feminist, indigenous, racial, and communitarian perspectives, which argue for the validation of 'other' knowledge and 'other' ways of knowing (Stacey, 1988; Kobayashi, 1994; Stanfield, 1994; Smith, 1999; Servaes, 1999; Tehranian, 1994; Sardar, 2002). These perspectives have long been demanding changes in existing frameworks, values and systems to bring marginalized experiences to the centre. The author draws support from these arguments in exploring the methodological possibilities that will guide me through

F. Malik, *Addressing Health Inequalities through Community Media*,
https://doi.org/10.1007/978-3-031-35237-9_3

the maze of literature on feminism, post-structuralism and liberation theology to develop a non-essentialist framework. This seems an uncertain outline but this work is not about certainties. The study is a challenge to formal and accepted foundations, which demands a high degree of reflexivity and strong political commitment. Lather (1991) argues that engaging within an uncertain framework emerges as the 'hallmark of liberatory praxis in a time marked by the dissolution of authoritative foundations of knowledge' (1991, p. 13). Adopting this approach to work through this methodological intricacy opens up ways for thinking outside the disciplinary rigidities and essentialist reading of various perspectives to develop productive philosophical reflections.

As we have seen in the first chapter of this thesis, the actions taken to address the process of social exclusion are not very different from the process of developmentalism used in the 'Third World'. One striking features of these discourses is the disregard shown to local knowledge and experience (Melkote & Steeves, 2001). The modernisation inspired model of pumping money and reliance on technology has not brought much qualitative change in many poor parts of the world.

This study underlines the importance of experiential learning, supported by the cultural practices of the marginalized people. The concept of increasing the individual's awareness of oppression and accompanying it with actions as suggested by Freire (1974), links the social aspects of life with the spiritual and vice versa. In doing so, the framework disproves the belief that social research is an objective, clinical and the value-free way of understanding humans, their relations and realities. Lather (1991) locates this framework at the 'conjunction of the feminisms, neo-Marxism and poststructuralism', to see how research and pedagogy could be 'positioned as fruitful sites' within a 'postmodern praxis' (1991, p. 11) Critical theory, feminism and liberation theology share the reasoned perspective on existing social injustice, collective social action and outlining empowering substitutes to existing structures.

Whether interested in individual, social or communal empowerment, these perspectives critique the capitalist system. Melkote and Steeves (2001) bring three perspectives closer by defining development within liberation theology as a 'process of liberation from injustice, discrimination and oppression'. Despite some similarities, there is a resistance to collaboration between these areas. Rejection of religion, call to revolution and the emphasis on institutions rather individuals in Marxist thinking are some of the major disagreements it has with liberation theology (Turner, 1994; Zweig, 1991).

As was discussed at some length in Chap. 2, modernization-led discourse sees progress as a process of secularization, and the 'unspoken assumption is that economic aid addresses material needs, whereas religion speaks primarily to spiritual needs that may be in conflict with material gain' (Melkote & Steeve, 2001: 274). Marxist thought more explicitly sees religion as more problematic, 'opiate of the masses', blinding people to material inequalities and injustice. With more interest being shown in the empowerment paradigm, especially in the local culture, knowledge and community based local grass roots movements, more emphasis is being laid on the context in which people live. Religion, culture and community life is seen as significant part of this context. This new paradigm of development tries to overcome old barriers between secular and profane and where various conflicting perspectives come together in a creative way to address issues of marginalisation, oppression and dispossession.

John H. Stanfield, writing from an Afro-American experience, seeks to de-Europeanise approaches in order to develop ethnic models of qualitative research. Stanfield argues that the 'ethnic modeling in qualitative research must involve questioning the knowledge' that researchers of European descent have been legitimising and calls for serious critique of Western methods and methodologies in order to develop alternative ways of knowing and doing things (1994:183). The need for liberating methodologies is more particularly urgent because 'colonization of knowledge' is seen not only as domination by the West over knowledge but also the ways and means to acquire and claim it. Linda Tuhiwai Smith, exploring the intersections of imperialism, knowledge and research, writes that 'the West has assumed the role of an archive of knowledge and systems, rules and values to determine research agendas, models and criteria' (1999: 42–43). Quoting Stuart Hall's analysis of 'the West' as a process of classification, a system of representation, a model of comparison and a criterion of evaluation, she argues that Western research is more than just research that is located in a positivist tradition (Hall, 1992a, b:259). Melkote and Steeves (2001: 198) quoting Braidotti (1994) sympathise with the alternative vision and share a common theme in critiquing the Western development discourse for the 'violence inflicted upon local, non-Western indigenous way of life and call for the recovery of dominated people's subjugated knowledge'. Coinciding with the demands for reconceptualisation of knowledge-gathering ways is the change taking place in the area of humanities as the accepted boundary between disciplines and their recognised methods are also being contested. Concepts such as race, gender and sexuality that have emerged as a result of this transformation have encouraged interdisciplinary approaches.

David Lloyd (1999: 3) attributes this change to 'the philosophical and theoretical critique of Western culture from within' and the return of 'social types and cultures' that were subjugated by the modernity project. He underlines the importance of decolonizing and other social movements in this process:

> *Consequently, the conjunction and intersection of immanent and returning critical movements have posed a profound intellectual challenge to the presumed universality of Western knowledge and deployed alternative theoretical approaches that can no longer be disavowed or looked down upon. In general, the new formations of knowledge that have arisen out of these conjunctions require interdisciplinary approaches and take for their objects phenomena which do not easily belong within the purview of traditional disciplinary terrains. In fact, they are usually not to be defined by a specific object at all but by their study of the processes of object construction – gendering, radicalization, cultural formations, for example – as these take place at the intersections of disciplines and social practices. This emphasis on the processes of representation and contestation in the construction of cultures and subjects puts in question the possibility and status of universal validity as a goal of the human as well as the natural sciences.* (Lloyd, 1999: 3–4)

This shift in social practice along with a contemporary desire for a less centralised and more participatory society is taking place at a time when people especially religious, ethnic and linguistic groups living as minorities in different parts of the world are becoming more assertive about who they are, and demanding a legitimacy of their way of life (Samad, 2004). This change has encouraged an overlapping of theories and perspectives where certainties and rigidities are constantly being eroded by possibilities and flexibilities. Many Muslim scholars influenced by critical theory are now talking about a new hegemony questioning both Marxism and religious bigotry (Sardar, 2002). A deviation can also be seen within Marxism and feminism as many followers of these standpoints do at times differ from their peers to recognise the importance of religion and spirituality in confronting racial, gender and class discrimination. In her thought provoking study on the education of Muslim girls, Kaye Haw, illustrates this multiplicity of feminism and sympathises with the religious needs of the girls to be taught in Islamic schools (Haw, 1998). Thus, despite the differences across different perspectives, there are shared concerns and solidarities that can lead to co- operations and reciprocal impression, in which scholars like Kellner (2001:3) see a possibility of 'productive synthesis' of critical theory and philosophy of liberation.

The overall tone of this work demands an analysis that engages with, and challenges the types of social organization through a sustained inquiry into the relationships between language, subjectivity and power which bring feminism and poststructuralism closer. Weedon (1997: 20) suggests the framework of 'feminist poststructuralism' for articulating a 'particular position and method' which addresses the 'question of how social power is exercised and how social relations of gender, class and race might be transformed'. Influenced by Michael Foucault's concern with history and his work on discourse and power, Weedon (Ibid) sees subjectivity and consciousness as critical for change:

> Through a concept of discourse which is seen as a structuring principle of society, in social institutions, modes of thought and individual subjectivity, feminist poststructuralism is able, in detailed, historically specific analysis, to explain the working of power on behalf of specific interests and to analyse the opportunities of resistance to it. It is a theory which decenters the rational, self-present subject of humanism, seeing subjectivity and consciousness socially produced in language, as sites of struggle and potential change. Language is not transparent as in humanist discourse; it is not expressive and does not label a 'real' world. Meanings do not exist prior to their articulation in language and language is not abstract system, but is always socially and historically located in discourses. Discourses represent political interests and in consequence are constantly vying for status and power. The site of this battle for power is the subjectivity of the individual and it is a battle in which the individual is an active bit not sovereign protagonist. (1997: 40)

Feminism and poststructuralism, however, are neither singular concept nor do they collapse, irreversibly, into a homogenous theory. These perspectives tactically intersect and createspaces for understanding the composite effects of the interaction between self, gender, race and class (King, 1988). By engaging in social critical power (Fraser & Nicholson, 1993: 428) of feminism, poststructuralism not only brings theory closer to practice, but also offers unique insights into the area of social exclusion and marginalisation which is the primary concern of this thesis. Through this intersection, the framework helps to analyse the construction of meaning, power relationships, and the social and historical role of language on the debate on social exclusion/inclusion. This way the framework offers the means through which marginalization of particular groups can be uncovered by delving into the hierarchies of power that construct our realities (Kamler et al., 1994). Similarly, a body of scholarship is emerging from the intersection of religious studies and new perspectives in feminism, offering new frameworks grounded in experiential knowledge gathered in different social, cultural and spiritual contexts. Feminism is adapting to more pluralistic meanings and is in creative dialogue with other perspectives to engage with wider issues and injustices in the society. Poststructural feminism, postmodern feminism, post-feminism, along with feminist theology are some of the ways feminism is now engaging with other streams of scholarship to address the issues of racism, classism, colonialism and militarism, besides patriarchy which remains its core concern. Also, the concept of praxis in liberation theology and experience in feminism brings these two perspectives even closer as both believe in the inseparability of theory from practice (Bjorkgren, 2004).

Feminism, as one of the most vociferous supporters of learning from experience, especially of those marginalized, advocates an integrative, trans-disciplinary approach to knowledge which grounds theory contextually in the concrete realm of womens everyday lives (Stacey, 1988: 21). This empathy with the experiences of the marginalized is shared by racial, ethnic, communitarian and libertarian theories, which not only overcome the duality and positivism but offer framework(s) that ground marginalized experience as a valid counter to the hegemonic paradigm.

Feminist Perspectives

Feminist scholars believe that the world is socially constructed and they reject the value-free nature of research (Haig, 1997). The research model of feminist inquiry is critical and emancipatory, and it recognises reality, science and research within this context (Stanley & Wise, 1993). These scholars argue that traditional research has failed to engage with the life and experience of women, marginalizing many aspects of their existence. The inability of the quantitative methods to reflect the experiences of women has led feminists to support qualitative research, which is understood to facilitate a fuller expression of experiences. Jayartne and Stewart say that methods must permit respondents to describe the world as they experience it:

> *We must not do away with them by taking advantage of our privileged speaking to construct a sociological version, which we then impose upon them as their reality. We may not rewrite the other's world or impose upon it a conceptual framework, which extracts from it what fits ours. Our conceptual procedures should be capable of explicating and analysing the properties of their experienced world rather than administering it. Their reality, their varieties of experience must be an unconditioned datum.* (1991: 93)

This approach of making methodology and methods integral parts of knowledge creation through increased participation of stakeholders is fundamental not only to feminism but to a variety of other critical and liberation perspectives, which also support the validation of subjective knowledge', and underline the importance of overcoming 'dichotomies in theory and practice'. Feminism is widely accepted to have made a major contribution to research methodology through its critique of neo-positivism. Feminism questioned the divide between object and subject and displaced positivist rigidities to create space for the 'personal'. Raghuram et al. (1998) go further to suggest that present day critical research owes a great deal to the insightful reviews of empirical and interpretive knowledges influenced by the perspectives of feminism. Believed to be a politics to fight injustice and inequality as well as a set of theories to understand patriarchy and the possibilities of change, feminism generally sees theory and practice as one. Theory informs the feminist practice and the practice helps to develop theories of understanding voice, subjectivity and power relations. Weedon (1997) explaining this process from the feminist poststructuralism point of view says:

> *Most feminists assume an integral relationship between theory and practice. Starting from the politics of the personal, in which womens' subjectivities and experiences of everyday life become the site of the redefinition of patriarchal meanings and values of resistance to them. Feminism generates new theoretical perspectives from which the dominant can be criticized and new possibilities envisaged.* (1997: 5)

This study finds resonance with feminist criticism of conventional methodology as simplistic (Farrow, 1974), racist (Unger 1983), exploitative (Stanley & Wise, 1993) and positivist (England, 1993). This approach problematises the concept of community as unstable and unpredictable (Katz, 1994) and deconstructs the 'essentialist and universalist notion of race and femininity' (Kobayashi, 1994), and in place of conventional methodology, it recognizes contextual methodologies, open to the emotions and experiences of the marginalized (Nielsen, 1990: 6). Feminist research has been influenced by and has influenced many different branches of scholarship. The post-modern and poststructuralist questioning of universal truths and arguments which claim that knowledge is constructed, situated, partial and historically specific has further stimulated the debate, which is suspicious of objective foundations of knowledge. Patti Lather (1991), accepting these influences, has coined the word post-positivist to describe the alternative, emancipatory and subjective research practice.

Western feminism itself has fragmented and transformed mainly due its critique by women from poor countries and women of colour who argue that it 'discursively colonizes the material and historical heterogeneities of lives in the 'Third World' countries by taking a taking a 'monolithic notion of patriarchy' (Mohanty, 2003:19) and simplistic understanding of non-Western women as 'composite singular Third World woman' (Melkote & Steeves, 2001: 53). Feminists from the 'Third World' have criticised such assumptions as 'ethnocentric, even racist and irrelevant to their concerns' Spivak 1988. Similarly, Fraser and Nicholson (1990), arguing that questions of racism and classism are not addressed within Western feminism, write:

> *In recent years, poor and working-class women, women of colour, and lesbians have finally won a wider hearing for their objections to feminist theories which fail to illuminate their lives and address their problems. They have exposed the earlier quasi-meta-narratives, with their assumptions of universal female dependence and confinement to the domestic*

sphere, as false extrapolations from the experience of the white, middle-class, heterosexual women who dominated the beginnings of the second wave. (1990: 33)

This critique has led to debates over 'voice', 'visibility', 'silence' and so on as non -Western women, particularly from the 'Third World' countries, felt that disempowerment and dispossession can be felt by those who experience them. The resulting feminist epistemologies which stress the importance of situated knowledge and the coherence of feminist experience have, however, come under attack from postmodern feminists, who question the concrete womens' experience on which the knowledge can be built on (Benhabib, 1995). As a result of this critique, many feminist accept a more relational standpoint, rather than one based exclusively on women's experiences (Andermahr et al., 1997). The existence of multiple experiences and other forms of subjugation, stress the need to look at the discrimination of women in a wider context of other systems and structures of domination, including racism, homophobia and colonialism (Hill, 2000).

These critiques, realizations and subsequent engagements within emancipatory perspectives have led to the theorising emancipatory potential of social research. Within these perspectives the positivist paradigm is questioned and alternative methodologies and epistemologies are developed which help to explore alternative ways of knowing and doing (See Stanley and Wise, 1993). These challenges and changes have lead to the recognition of more than one way and level of analysis within this scholarship. We now talk about feminism(s) in the plural illustrating multiplicity in meanings and interpretations. This has also brought concepts of reflexivity, self-awareness and self-criticism into the area and acceptance of plurality and diversity within this scholarship. Reflecting upon its own notions, many scholars within feminism accept that there is no one feminist position.

These scholars have also ridiculed the idea of gender or class having a universalizing approach with a 'meta-narrative' within a 'totalizing discourse'. These scholars propose a historically contextualised and critical theory that recognises the cultural diversities and differences between women. These scholars, seen as postmodernist or poststructuralist feminists, highlight the need to move away from an essentialist concept of self to a complexly constructed and dynamic self (Fraser, 1995; Weedon, 1997). Despite these self- reflections, criticism and strategic coalitions with other scholarship, gender and gendered relations remain the main focus of feminism(s). The debates have made a significant impact on the way the counter discourse understands and validates the struggles of minorities, indigenous people and subjugated groups in relation to the powerful majority, institutionalised mainstream and hegemonic elite. Some scholars working within a communitarian perspective stress the need to learn from the diversity of womens' experiences and build coalitions as a 'political tool for interventions and action' based on common context of struggles against the oppression by gender, class, race, ethnicity, and nation, including colonisation (Steeves, 1993; 222). Standpoint feminism, which argues that the practice of feminism should reflect the standpoint of women (Hill, 2000) invites many scholars and students outside the perspective of feminism to draw support to their perspectives from feminism. Standpoint feminism helps them to theorise subjective knowledge by engaging in critical thought, action and reflection about experience, knowledge and relationship with social and political structures.

Although much of feminist thought shows solidarity with marginal people, their subjugated knowledge and experiences, it is the feminist geographers 'analysis of space and place which helps to analyse the discourse of social exclusion within inner-city areas. This is important for this study because of its focus on the immigrant community from South Asia who live in large clusters within the inner city Nottingham. This spatial significance brings with it debates on social deprivation and economic disadvantage on the one hand, and communal solidarity and cultural advantage on the other. Quoting Heidi Nast's work on the contributions feminist geographers have made in highlighting the importance of place in everyday construction of gender, recognition of difference among women and redefining of research field as a dynamic subjective space, Madge et al. (1997: 86) write that there are certain key characteristics in 'ways of knowing, ways of asking, ways of interpreting and ways of writing' which are central to feminist methodologies.

They argue that these approaches are not 'exclusive' or 'discrete' but create a process which is 'open to critique, reflection and debate.' The argument that womens' own interpretation of identities, experiences and power relations is crucial lends support to the author's argument that the knowledge and experience of marginalized minorities can offer a valid analysis of their situation. Harding (1991, 1998) argues that this positional advantage, which marginalized groups use to experience things differently, can help in raising a new set of research questions though she stresses one need not to be part of a marginalized group to raise such questions. In this study, the 'epistemic privilege' is crucial to the author as a researcher and the people he works with. The author is both a participant and subject while people in the community set the agenda for this research. This arrangement is only possible within a dynamic and flexible position. It helps the author to immerse himself in the life of the community and for the community to validate their subjective experience. The author see himself in all these roles all the time, as he takes the role of a presenter on Radio Ramzan, a listener to debates about inequality, an investigator asking questions and an observer of a process. It would be difficult to be all these in the absence of the 'privilege' which this framework offers me.

Poststructuralist Perspectives

It is important for a theory to be useful to explain how social power is used and how this power is structured around gender, class and race. Poststructuralism influenced by the structural linguistics, theory of difference, deconstruction theory, concept of ideology, psychoanalytical theories and discourse of power, shares some basic notions about 'language, meaning and subjectivity' (Weedon, 1997:13). It focuses on the primacy of theory, decentering of the subject, and the importance of the reader over the text to highlight the multiplicity and rearrangement of meaning (Sarup, 1988).

For this study this approach lends support to an analysis of the construct of social exclusion as an overlapping discourse of politics, bureaucracy, media and academic study and how those problematised are initiated into a counter- discourse informed by their own knowledge, experience and world-view to offset the discourse of the dominant. Within this counter discourse, peoples' reference to faith, culture and their experiences of immigration and racism are evaluated as a set of discursive practices. The thesis draws support from the arguments that knowledge about the social world is created through shifting patterns of discourses in which and through which meanings are shaped (Hollway, 1984; Davis, 1993).

Foucault sees discourse as the site and contestation of power in which processes, regulations, and structures, along with resistances and oppositions interplay to shape meaning and represent the 'normal'. Power is central to the Foucauldian concept of discourse. He sees power as relational and not 'simply repressive' and suggests that power can only be said to 'create an effect if the object of power has the ability to resist' (Sheridan, 1980: 217). This way Foucault provides a tool which can explain how power is exercised through discourse and how resistance is possible against this exercise. Foucault's work on homosexuality and femininity illustrates how problematization incites discourse which leads to counter discourse: as homosexuality stands up and speaks on its own to demand its legitimacy and naturality. So these problematizations create hurdles, which are contested and resisted. Similarly, in the context of the use of the female body, Foucault argued that the process of the sexual exploitation of women led feminist movements to define and legitimise their own worldview by reinventing their 'own type of existence, political, economic and cultural' (Kristsman, 1990: 115).

Escobar (1992, 1995) has taken up the Foucauldian turn in development studies, identifying development discourse as a series of statements and 'visibilities' linked together as a chart of power. Development within this perspective is seen as the cartography of power and knowledge. Along these lines, the understanding of power is the overarching theme of this work. In order to analyse the complexity and interrelatedness of power relations, this framework allows me as a researcher to engage with the discourses through review and self-critique to appreciate the correlation of power-sensitive perspectives. Foucault's discourse analysis also lends support to theorizing the highly complex construct of community as a series of discursive relationships consisting of a number of shifting perspectives of race, ethnicity, religion, politics and immigration. There are voices within the voiceless as there are peripheries and centres among the marginalized. This study accepts the differences and similarities and acknowledges the inequalities within the unequal as a set of discursive relationships. While the minority ethnic groups may be discriminated against on the basis of ethnicity, minority status, immigration status, colour of the skin, nevertheless within these discriminated groups, women, disabled people and homosexuals are also treated unequally.

This dynamic conceptualisation of subject positions lends support to the authors' theorisation of community as a fluid and strategic positioning of various subjectivities. As is explained in detail in Chap. 4 of this thesis, the members of Mirpuri community become black, ethnic, minority, immigrant and non-white on one hand and Muslim, Pakistani, Kashmiri, Sunnis, Barailves etc. on the other. This way some labels and subject positions are used tactically and those subjectified became part of the process of subjectification.

This recognition of fragmentations and diversity within the research field highlights the need to take the different contexts and participants 'multiple, shifting and contradictory discourses and subjectivities' into account when we construct the marginalized. On the whole, this study engages with a multifaceted network of relationships, associations and contestations, which demonstrate varying levels of power, influence and impact. This power is not fixed but changes as situations and contexts change. Within the structure of Radio Ramzan, the power of the management committee over scheduling and topics, the power of listeners to walk into the studio and make their point and above all their power to turn the radio off, combined with the power of the presenter to make, influence and challenge opinions and public perceptions, the power of the Radio Authority[1] to monitor the content and set guidelines, and the power of sponsors to support the radio, all form a myriad of power relations.

Within the community, power relations between various tribes, kinships, various shades of religious thought, country of origin, status, age, and gender all create a maze of power relations. These relations are very dynamic and come into play in different ways, and can prove as enablement as well as constraint; productive as well negative (Lukes, 1974; Foucault, 1972, 1979). This subjectivity as theorised within the poststructuralist thought is a constantly changing positioning related with others (Davies, 1993), and it opens up the possibility of accepting or rejecting from a number of different subject positions within different discourses and contexts. This subjectivity is not always self-proclaimed, but can also be the result of how the individual is positioned and subjectified by others. Hence subjectivity is a dynamic process in which the individual becomes an active agent (Lowe, 1998). Another aspect of power is the relationship between the researcher and the researched, and how this relationship becomes part of deriving meanings out of daily living experiences.

In this study, this aspect is very critical. The research question, the position, the objectives from this study, and the background of the researcher all create another set of discursive perspectives which become a 'producer of meaning' along with the perspectives of the researched in a collaborative process (Haw, 1998). The adaptation of a discursive framework is consistent with the epistemological position taken in this study, which walks away from simplicities, certainties and rigidities. Weedon (1997) argues that the feminist poststructuralist perspectives help to analyse the nature of power and subjective identity created through a variety of discourses to develop an alternate knowledge base. Barrett (1991), contextualising Foucault's work, suggests that the concept of discourse as an alternate theoretical model is based on the relational and dynamic concept of power, and not an absolute or static understanding of power.

Liberation Theology Perspective

As a third component of this analysis, the liberation theology perspective helps to create awareness about the voicelessness and how it can be addressed through what can be done about it by consciousness raising, reflection and action. The liberation point of view links 'spiritual growth and empowerment with material needs', and prefers' cultural and spiritual practices' in the process of empowerment (Melkote & Steeve, 2001: 296). By adopting a methodology in favour of the powerless and marginalized, the thesis creates a commonality with liberation theology. Knitter (1987), arguing for social and economic justice through the institutions of faith, writes:

> *If the religions of the world can recognise poverty and oppression as a common problem, if they share a common commitment to remove such evils; they will have a basis for reaching across their in commensurabilities and differences in order to hear and understand each other and possibly be transformed in the process.* (1987:186)

Liberation theology argues that the hope of surviving the conditions of disenfranchisement and marginalisation of people can be found within their own faith. This point of view makes the basic tenets of the Christian liberation theology which took root in Latin America in the early 1960's and preferred practice over doctrine (orthopraxis over orthodoxies) and favoured 'preferential option for the poor' (Gutiérrez, 1988). The Brazilian scholar Paulo Freire (1972) calls this process 'conscientization'. Freire, who brought concepts of empowerment and freedom from oppression into development discourse highlighting the role of human agency in the growth and progress of communities, introduced the notion of emancipatory development. This standpoint envisages a shift in power from external factors to 'individuals, organizations, and communities over social and economic conditions, over political processes and over their own stories' (Melkote & Steeves, 2001:366).

Liberation perspectives are close to the goals of this thesis, which explore the role cultural practices and faith can play in generating critical dialogue within a religious minority. Radio Ramzan, the community based radio station run within the religious ethos is used as a case study in this exploration. Liberation theology as theorized within the development communication scholarship foregrounds 'emancipatory communication' that could help people break free from existing models and structures to determine their own future. This means a dialogue rather a monologue, a horizontal, rather than vertical flow of communication, where the communicators and listeners change their roles. These dialogic processes are seen to 'enable participants to identify and explore issues' (Ibid: 365). Looking at the existing structure of media regulation in the UK, it reveals a strict duopoly, dominated by the commercial media on the one hand and public service the British Broadcasting Corporation (BBC). The critique of the public service broadcasting and the BBC's centrality in the current regulatory arrangement is well documented (Negrine, 1989).The current broadcasting scenario has come under scathing attacks and its 'traditionally established relationship with politics, culture and the audience, as a kind of domestic diplomatic service, representing the British – or what has been projected 'as the best of the British', at a time when 'middle class Britain is' seen at odds with divided Britain' (Lewis & Booth, 1989: 69). The current media structure is seen to have failed to represent this varied spectrum and tended to exclude or marginalize all those who stayed outside accepted central boundaries of political argument.

Here a Freirian analysis helps to theorise a community-based communal media that can give voice and platform for interaction and engagement. When used in conjunction with feminist and poststructural analysis, this framework opens up such possibilities. The methods of Participatory Action Research (PAR), which this thesis adopts to map the fieldwork, challenges practices that separate the researcher from the researched, promotes the forging of a partnership between researchers and the people under study. Both researcher and participant become actors in the investigative process, influencing the flow, interpreting the content, and sharing options for action.

The process of participatory research is seen as itself empowering because it forges togetherness, signifies context, legitimizes experience and transforms living knowledge into action. Thus participatory research reflects goal-oriented, experiential learning, and transformative pedagogy (Dewey, 1938; Mead, 1934; Freire, 1974). Within the alternative scholarship, there is a common ground emerging between various perspectives, which might have opposing principles but share a strategic position that allows them to engage creatively in addressing bigger challenges. Melkote and Steeves (2001) identifying these common grounds where liberation theology, feminism and Marxism can tactically meet, argue:

> *Just as Liberation theologies challenge religious traditions that emphasize spirituality without social awareness, many who identify with Marxism and Feminism deviate from their anti-religious peers by acknowledging the importance of spirituality as a resource for challenging class, gender, and other forms of oppression.* (2001: 293)

Black feminist theologians argue that liberation theology can become a dynamic process when it engages with feminism to address issues of marginality. These theologians base their arguments on their experience of finding the 'vernacular reading' of biblical texts, through the art of story-telling, empowering for the Dalits (low caste) women in India (Melanchthon, 2005). Though facing multiple discriminations as low caste poor Christian women in a cast-ridden, patriarchal and mainly Hindu nation, Dalit women are considered to be 'concerned not just for their own welfare, but for the welfare of their entire communities, their men, their sons and their daughters' (Ibid: 220).

This specific feminist hermeneutics practiced by the low caste Christian women in India is very different from the mainstream reading of the biblical texts, and these non-formal methods, emerging from the local culture and communication processes, help women to 'release themselves from andocentric interpretative processes, placing them side by side with their own experiences and identities' (Rebera, 1997:94). This way, when the oppressed understand scriptures through their own experiences and not through the eyes of their oppressors, the narrative of spirituality engages with the life stories of the oppressed, leading to a challenge to the oppression (Barton, 2005). The act of sharing spiritual thoughts personally, consciously and politically through the medium of stories can help the marginalized subjects to understand their position and develop agency to fight back through their own faith and cultural practices. For many excluded people who are discriminated against because of their background and social status, the use of such empowering and imaginative 'learning by doing' approach gives them both voice and power over their own stories. This approach is promoted within all types of feminisms and also forms the basis of Freire's concept of liberation theology.

Treading the Uncertain Path

By developing a methodology supported by various, at times conflicting, perspectives and approaches, the study seeks epistemological plurality to discover 'representational meaning', rather than to 'find explanations' through the deconstruction of the dominant ideology, 'acceptance of multiple meanings and strengthening consciousness' (Servaes, 1999; Tehranian 1994). So the thesis envisions processes that include exploration into social and cultural studies approaches to race, immigration and identity; development and policy studies approach to poverty and exclusion; and communication and theological approaches to empowerment and participation. These approaches, however, are not mutually exclusive but overlap and inter-weave as happens in real life. The growing interest in how emancipatory perspectives can create a contextual understanding of marginalised points of view has led to the discourse of 'hear the voice' to bring the marginal subject to the centre and give socially silenced group a voice which has otherwise remained stifled. These processes are seen more as forms of 'recognition' and not redistribution of materials resources (Fraser, 1995).

However, by conceptualizing agency and structure as interdependent and interacting, the actions do impact on institutions. Agency here means the faculty of individuals to act and do things that could affect the social relationships while 'structure' refers to the social institutions and provisions individuals find themselves in. While the structure-agency dualism dominates the social and political debate, this study goes beyond this dualism to suggest that action and structures are interdependent, and at times converge and overlap (Giddens, 1976). This thesis puts agency at the centre of the analysis to suggest how the members of the Mirpuri community can make a difference by validating their points of view through participation, reflection and action. This approach highlights the transformative capacity of power of the agency to affect the institutional power (Giddens, 1987). Agency, however, does not mean that power can shift altogether from the centre to peripheries but opens up the possibility of recognizing other realities where the marginalized can have an alternative vision of who they are. The thesis sees this vision as a process through which individuals, organisations and communities engage with their social and economic conditions and participate in their communal activities to take control over their stories.

Although feminism does not see agency and structure this way, it helps to expose the conditions that contribute to exploitation and patriarchy. This approach of feminist research lends support to the study in conceptualizing the community radio among the marginalized Mirpuri community as a platform upon which to act and reflect. This way of privileging marginalized experiences into actions through a variety of emancipating and liberating methods, helps their 'voice' enter into the research text. This is closer to the feminist standpoint theories of knowledge which highlight the proposition that women, due to their personal and social experience as females, are in a better position to understand their world (Stacey, 1988; Hill, 2000, Harding, 1998). Some scholars, however, argue that there are a variety of standpoints based on class, ethnicity, race, culture and education, but the supporters of standpoint theory believe that some common criteria guide theory and research in this context (Harding, 1998). Such a research approach helps to overcome the research/ researched and theory / practice divide. Through the prolonged action and interaction, the researcher and participants jointly construct this discourse.

By approaching the study in this subjective way, the author is aware that he may invite many questions on his position, the methodology and any claims the author makes make. The study is very explicit about being subjective in order to explore worldviews of those who remain marginalized. This approach, as argued earlier in this chapter draws support from feminism, poststructuralism and liberation theology to validate the experiential knowledge of the excluded people in a bid to facilitate the empowerment of these people from their own cultural practices. By engaging with these issues from the very beginning, The author acknowledges the significance of the context in which this work is carried out. It clarifies that any assertions and observations he makes are situated and partial. But this does not mean the arguments put forward in this study lack thoroughness and the framework adopted to analyze these arguments is invalid. The author believes that there is no boundary between the field of research and the authors own surroundings. The author does not switch on and off, and there is no '9–5' in this work. It does not start and stop. This is an ongoing process. In this process, theory and practice blend into the living experience.

So when the researcher looks at the fieldwork, he looks at certain aspects of his own life. His field diary reveals the overlapping and interconnectedness of living, working and studying. He does not invite the community members into office and give them closed questionnaires to fill in, but he chats with them while in the queue at the ASDA stores or while waiting for groceries shop or before and after prayers in the local mosque. This way of generating/gathering exploring knowledge in author's case is a natural, open and liberating way. Since such approaches see knowledge as experiential and contextual, many feminist scholars have found it appropriate for research from their standpoint because it encourages democratic relationship between the knower and known and rejects false dualisms (Stacey, 1988). The discursive rules and regulations of academia apply to the researcher and his work which eventually make him a researcher and eventually a writer. This process cannot be said to be impartial or neutral (Usher, 1996). By accepting 'reflexivity' in his research, the researcher acknowledge tha this position is implicated in a discursive practice.

A Dynamic Framework

The perspectives of feminism, post-structuralism and liberation theology, though different, share epistemological plurality and critique the modernism-influenced positivist research. These perspectives, as explained in earlier sections of this chapter, 'privilege' de-centered subjects through 'action and reflection', highlight the role of 'voice' and critical consciousness, question the 'essentialist concept of truth and knowledge' by offering possibilities 'other way of knowing and doing' and examine of the relation between 'other' and 'self' (Freire, 1972; Lather, 1991; Davis, 1993; Sardar, 1997; Haw, 1998; Kobayashi, 1994; Melkote & Steeves, 2001). This study embraces all the differences and commonalities which define the community and understands community more as a position rather than organic entity. Such a conceptualisation demands a framework which is non-deterministic and flexible enough to accommodate the diversity and dynamism of the field. However, bringing differing perspectives together can be problematic, but as mentioned before, this type of framework is closer to the broader aims of this thesis to question the pigeonholing of knowledge and compartmentalization of academic inquiry. The thesis draws support from the work of other scholars who have analysed complex social and cultural issues with the help of multi- perspective and inter-disciplinary approaches.

Kaye Haw (1998) analyzing contemporary discourses of race, religion, ethnicity, class and gender within a Muslim community over the issues of education within the state school system in Britain finds the feminist poststructuralist analysis attractive:

> *It provides a useful analytical tool capable of illuminating and revealing how power is exercised through discourse, how oppression works and how resistance might be possible. Also this is of direct relevance to the relationship between the researcher and the participants in any piece of research, allowing as it does for an understanding that both researcher and participants are active producers of meaning so that this has to be critically explored and placed within the text.* (1998:12)

In order to understand the politics of difference and commonality, Avtar Brah (1992) stresses working through the multiple configurations of power like gender, race, ethnicity, nationalism, generation and sexuality which she thinks signify the special type of power relations through which a variety of economic, political and cultural practices are articulated. Such study needs a multi-disciplinary approach in which paradigms, frameworks and insights enter into an engagement to create what she calls a 'creolised' envisioning (1992: 143). With regard to this research these perspectives and author's own position provide a kaleidoscope in which various points of view shift, compete, co-exist and change meaning so that experiences of community could be seen as a set of discursive relationships comprising various sometimes contradictory discourse such as race, culture, religion and media. The dynamism within feminism, Post-structuralism and the empowerment objectives of Liberation theology lends support to this framework but does not mean there is an absolute consistency within these perspectives. This argument runs parallel with the epistemology that the way to empathize with this subjective knowledge is to experience it. Since this is a dynamic process of creating, interpreting and living, it can best be observed rather than discovered in terms of empirical evidence. So methodologically, this demands moving out of laboratories into the real world to touch, feel and live this knowledge. In order to know it, one has to get involved. So in line with this epistemology, non-empirical methods of action research like participant observation can enhance this quality of meaning, interpretation and experience.

In feminism, self-reflexivity and empathy with the subjects is used to validate subjectivity. Within one of the earliest definitions of feminist social research: on, by and for women, formulated by Liz Stanley and Sue Wise (1993), it is argued that the subject position of the researcher, or producer of knowledge, produces better knowledge if she is politically committed. Maria Mies (1999) argues that feminist perspectives replace the value-free research of neutrality and indifference towards the research objects by conscious partiality. Although the thesis does not exclusively adopt a feminist methodological approach, it has many objectives which are very close to feminist critical aims.

The study adopts the characteristics of feminist methods in exploring discourses of social exclusion within the Mirpuri community, which comprises men, women and children. Raghuram et al. (1998) underline the important features of feminist research as those having emancipatory goals, validating the notion of subjectivity, being aware of ethics and being self-reflexive. Along with these commonalities with feminist research, this project is also informed by the post- structural understanding of relational power and discourse. This lends support to me to provide an insider's account of how this radio station provides a context for communicative interaction among the marginalized people to organise and engage in practices that help them to define their own worldview.

Similarly, Liberation theology through the process of conscientization (Freire, 1974) revitalizes the local knowledge base by reviving indigenous and marginalized existence. These perspectives recognise faith, culture and tradition by acknowledging the role of spirituality in empowering people. Such empowerment based on a way of life is seen to increase the effectiveness within grass roots movements. With its focus on the Mirpuri community living in inner city Nottingham, the study is built on the epistemological ground that life experience structures one's understanding of life. This worldview is seen by many scholars to play a significant role in the re-conceptualization of knowledge and development to displace the Western worldview, although it is in itself by no means unproblematic. Sardar, indicating the 'power shift towards a non-Western way of doing things argues that 'there will be more than one dominant way of being human, of being free, and there will be more than one way to develop' (Sardar, 1997:47).

This study particularly looks at how, through communal interaction on the community- based radio, the kinship networks, religious customs, and cultural practices help in increasing the participation and empowerment of individuals and the community as a whole. The study is carried out as participatory action research actively involved in knowledge production through 'engagement, education, communication, action and reflection' (Finn, 1994: 27). This approach lends support to an analysis which challenges the institutionalized mass media from small-scale community-based initiatives. The initiatives that are grass roots based and which encourage horizontal rather than vertical patterns of mass media. This framework makes it possible to actively involve the author to increase the participation of community members in the radio project which facilitates a two-dimensional communication in which sender and receiver are involved in a 'dynamic process; that could lead to social action (McQuail, 1994).

The Shifting Patterns of the Author's Position

This project is an outcome of interaction between a number of perspectives, which include author's story, his experience and his politics. His position, though central to the study, nevertheless raises many questions. Before the author goes on to explore how he is positioned in this study, it is worth mentioning here that the author does not see 'himself' as a monolithic and coherent entity. His gender, age, profession, background, language, knowledge and perceptions create 'conflicting' tensions and knowledge claims. In order to carry out this study, he needed to explore how these multiple concepts of self-engage with various dimensions of this study, especially the subjects who also are many things at many times.

The author argues that such approach is vital in building space for marginalized voices which otherwise remain stifled within institutionalized spaces and processes. Working, participating and living with minority groups and experiencing a marginalized existence, he is a victim, a witness and observer of a discourse which excludes people by 'othering' them their way of life, their knowledge, and at times, putting the blame of disadvantage on the disadvantaged. But he is also a witness to a counter discourse through which marginalized people engage in communicative interaction, draw strength from their culture and create communal spaces of resistance to assert their way of life. So, his first-hand experience is central to both these processes. Marilyn Nisaam Sabat (2002) in a moving autobiographical account of her experience mentions how she explored the dimensions of political activism, feminism, philosophy and spirituality to understand the process of victim blaming in the US:

> *As I have developed in the decades since all of these dimensions have become central to my existence, I have at the same time felt more and more deeply disturbed by the continuance and intensification of anti-black and other racisms, including anti-Semitism, backlash against women, gays, and immigrants in this country and elsewhere in the world, and by the growing dominance of global capital. In my struggle to comprehend these things, I have come to see that victim-blaming is one of the most significant, if not the most significant, mechanism perpetuating our failure to create a more just, humane environment for all*

people. (Victim-blaming includes blame by perpetrators, self-blame by victims, and blame by public opinion.) For as long as victim-blaming pervades our lives, for so long we will be deflected from focusing on understanding the origins of the unnecessary suffering we inflict on ourselves and others. But that is not all. In addition, we will be deflected from doing anything constructive even where the origins of suffering are identified. In my struggle to understand victim-blaming, a phenomenon everywhere in evidence yet profoundly difficult to comprehend, I have found it necessary to try to develop a synthesis of feminist, philosophical, and spiritual resources. (2002: 270)

Living, working and researching within the community gives the author insights into it but he cannot claim that there are no barriers or inhibitions, as 'complete participation in the situation is impossible; such immersion would risk going native, and so a degree of marginality in the situation is needed to do research' (Walsh, 2000: 233). The community is a highly complex and problematic concept, and he see his relationship with the heterogeneous community as dynamic. By declaring his politics and intentions, he share the space and sentiment for the validation of knowledge, giving a voice and raising awareness. For these reasons the methodological and epistemological questions are of paramount importance and are deeply connected. This relationship can be best explained through participatory action research. However, the author does not claim the knowledge generated and recorded through the methodology is the only knowledge but he accept it as one of the realities in the multiplicity of realities that determine the 'other'.

The author is conscious of the fact that his thesis engages with a fund of literature from feminist perspectives, which demands a greater level of reflexivity on his part and the need to be self-critical. As a heterosexual man, working in a male dominated environment, he should be conscious of the fact not to pick and choose concepts but to engage with different shades and opinions within the feminist discourse. From the research question to the author's preferred methodology and methods, this study is naturally attracted towards emancipatory perspectives, especially the perspective of women and their politics. Although this study is not a feminist project as such, feminism offers a variety of ways of looking at things that guide me through the theorising the marginalisation of the members of the Mirpuri community. Feminist research emphasizes that different positions and situations give different meanings to the understanding of the world, and different realities between the researcher and researched need to be explicated as part of research analysis. Raghuram et al. (1998:39) emphasize this relationship by arguing that 'researchers are part of the social world and their positions within this world, their experiences and their ethical commitments inform both their work and their research'.

While gender has been the primary basis for feminist critiques of epistemological and methodological practices, there has been a growing emphasis upon how racial and ethnic difference shapes the relationship between the researcher and the researched. For me, working and living in the community was an advantage and, secondly, the work was directly related with the community development. Radio Ramzan the community-based communication project was an integral part of this process, and the author was associated with the licensing, setting up and programming of this station. However, to declare author as a researcher doing 'research within his own community' has been a very difficult decision. Being an action research project, the author's 'activeness' in the project is both a hurdle and a potential.

With these dilemmas in mind, the author owns this research as a subjective view of the world the author lived in. The framework for analysis of fieldwork uses a methodology which is dynamic and one evolved from multiple disciplines. This multi- disciplinary approach involves competing standpoints to look at fieldwork from multiple visions. These visions are vital in studying the diversity of the 'field' since the research space is an arena of differences and similarities. The 'field' of study is the community in which the author lives, work and experience marginalisation and struggles to overcome it. This space is not a neutral or homogenous area but a social and political construct where similarities and diversities co-exist. The people in question are a Muslim population comprised mostly of the people of Pakistani/Mirpuri origin living in inner city Nottingham. People themselves take control of the process of emancipation, which recognizes the importance of Participatory Action Research (PAR) in initiating collaborative social action. Having ownership of the process, the methodology itself is empowering for local knowledge as participants develop their own methods of raising consciousness followed by reflection, leading to participatory social action.

The author consciously take a particular epistemological position, where he accept fieldwork as situated and partial. But this situatedness is explicit and partiality is conscious, highlighting the fact that knowledge and power relations influence this study. The critique of modernisation and its Western, white, masculine agenda has fore- grounded the debate about who researches whom and with what agenda. Many black analysts including Carby (1982) and Collins (1990) argue that issues around race have been neglected by white researchers, and that the findings by white researchers may not apply to ethnic minority groups or may misrepresent them. By writing about his own experience, the author's position becomes an integral part of this study. The author makes clear in this research questions that the thesis is more of subjective appraisal based on his interpretation. This interpretation is not one based on detached data analysis in a controlled laboratory situation but an engaged experiential real life understanding.

The research takes into account not just what transpires in conversations but explores the contexts in which these conversations take place. When the author convers with a taxi driver, the conversation takes place in a taxi, and author can identify with some of the experiences of the driver. The authors detailed radio listening as part of participant observation in the taxi of driver QA, while he is waiting for passengers at the Nottingham train station, exposes me to unique perspectives which are only accessible by a position that overcomes the researcher/researched divide. Similarly, having a meal at the Royal Sweets shop on Gregory Boulevard in Hyson Green makes the author feel part of an extended family where everyone knows everyone else. With the evening show of the radio in the background, eating with friends helps the author get a feedback which is spontaneous and immediate. Understanding daily living experiences of the members of Mirpuri community, and exploring the impact of these experiences on their social, cultural and spiritual life forms an essential part of his engagement. The research, therefore, is directed at the understanding as well as the transformation of social realities of these people, and Radio Ramzan provides a dynamic context for such insights and the QA would often drive the author home via the train station and give him, at times, unsolicited feedback on radio shows, and share his views on 'community politics'.

Exploring Experiences Through PAR

Participatory action research (PAR), which evolved out of the liberationist ideas of Paulo Freire, is explicitly political in nature with the overt objectives of restoring oppressed peoples' 'ability to create knowledge' and practice in their own interests. As a process of exploring subjugated knowledge, PAR facilitates dialogue to 'empower, motivate, increase self-esteem, and develop community solidarity' (Becker & Bryman, 2004: 118). These objectives can be located in various critical and emancipatory perspectives which emphasise 'enabling', 'empowerment' and 'giving voice' to the marginalised, putting research capabilities in their hands so that they can identify themselves as knowing actors; defining reality, shaping identity, naming history and transforming lives (Callaway, 1992; Fernandes & Tandon, 1981; Humphries & Truman, 1994; Stanley & Wise, 1993). Without going into grand theories to provide universal analysis, the participatory perspectives have their focus on people, an endogenous vision of development and attention to issues of power and equality.

Participatory action research thus brings the theoretical framework developed in the earlier part of this chapter into life by offering the means to realize the objectives of this thesis in a non-essentialist and the non-positivist way. When applied to Radio Ramzan, PAR helps to open debates and facilitate participation of stakeholders by providing a platform to 'identify issues; to reclaim a sense of community and emphasize the potential for liberation; and to make sense of information collected' (Reason, 1994: 239). By way of summary we would emphasize that action research is not a methodology but an orientation that shapes methodological practices. There are no right answers, rather lots of choices, and the quality of inquiry is shaped by the appropriateness of these choices and the way they are made (Becker & Bryman, 2004: 118).

So, instead of conceptualising research as detached discovery and empirical verification of generalizable patterns in community practice, the study explores research methodologies through which community practitioners mobilize information and knowledge resources, as one part of their broader strategies for community empowerment. This approach explores emancipatory methodologies under a political research agenda to validate, share and learn from experiences. The study demands a holistic approach, which puts observations and interview data into a larger perspective wherein human behaviour could be understood within the context of human life. Ethnography relies on personal experience and 'possible participation, not just observation' and using a variety of 'historical, observational, and interview methods', creating a 'narrative description of emerging and shifting research problems, perspectives, and theories' (Genzuk, 2003:1). Usually members of the group observed or studied have a strong sense of solidarity with each other, based on common factors of language, residence, social relationship, and religious and political beliefs and practices. This commonality facilitates the in- depth understanding of group dynamics, especially when the group is a minority and living or aspiring to live differently from the majority. The study argues that marginalised people are in a better position to identify and discuss their problems and have the capacity to address these problems. Participatory Action Research (PAR) evolved as a reaction to the intellectual domination of Western social research over the development process and this participatory and inclusive means empowers disadvantaged people to find answers within their community, taking cognizance of their social and cultural realities (Fals-Borda, 1979; Freire, 1972).

The study is based on a dynamic relationship between researcher and subjects, and it works towards the recovery of unity in research and practice. There are multiple collaborators and influences that have shaped this work. The primary collaborators of this process are the listeners (predominantly the members of Mirpuri community) of Radio Ramzan in Nottingham. As a participatory project, the influence of these people is of paramount importance in developing a holistic and qualitative description of their worldviews. The thesis has revolved around their experiences, practices and perspectives. While exploring these worldviews, the thesis has changed in focus, shape and design to allow the subjects to influence its content, conjecture and conclusions. Besides these known and unknown listeners of Radio Ramzan, the study has learnt from the daily interactions with five Mirpuri volunteers (presenters/producers) of Radio Ramzan whose hopes and fears, aspirations and realities are reflected throughout this study.

Their take on the social, political, cultural and spiritual issues pertinent to their 'marginalised lives' has made substantial part of this work. Besides these volunteers, the presence of a Mirpuri speaking, British-born, and highly political health worker on the HEAP Project has helped in putting in practice the various theories of health promotion and empowerment. Her consistent support and critical reflections on debates and discussions have helped in the introspection and evaluation of this work. In this regard, Chambers (1997, 2001) stresses the enabling of rural people to plan and enact solutions to problems by analysing their own knowledge of local conditions. This approach argued by some critical anthropologists to be borrowed from social anthropology, explicates participatory research methodologies as flexible art.

Participation is believed to have an inherent value for participants, particularly in addressing the issues of marginalisation and powerlessness, and it helps to adopt local/indigenous knowledge and experiences to address these issues. However, many argue that participation is not an absolute concept, and scholars have put forward a nuanced pattern of participation, ranging from passive participation to self-mobilization. Although the term participation is understood to be in the development discourse since 1950s (Rahnema 1992), it gained currency when participatory research methods were used to enhance the role for local people and their knowledge in various development initiatives. Chambers' work on participatory rural appraisal is thought to have gained increasing relevance as people with little skills were encouraged to express their knowledge and use their experience. But this approach and its tools have been mostly used within the positivist paradigm. The later use of participatory action research (PAR), which was developed against the notion of the neutrality of research (Fals-Borda & Rahman, 1991), led to community- driven development (CCD) to put the communities and the stakeholders in control of the development initiatives. All these efforts, however have neglected the dialogic use of communication necessary for making these initiatives successful. Freire, as a practitioner and scholar, actually developed the idea of empowerment through awareness of 'conscientization' to raise the awareness among the powerless about their conditions through an active process of reflection, action and dialog.

Within this framework, the study as an 'empowered dialogue', as conceptualized by Freire (1972, 1974) works at various levels. It not only facilitates people to participate but it works beyond the radio station in the community as context to celebrate and validate a way of life. The author's role role in this participatory action research project demands a constant dialogue, and as such, the study becomes a dynamic dialogue between a number of perspectives, and the author draws upon a combination of written, oral and nonverbal communication, emanating from a variety of interpersonal and group communications in the design, implementation and documentation of the research. The fieldwork, thus, draws upon various social research methods: unstructured in-depth interviews, focus group interviews, observation, archival and library research, and historical investigation, using documents and personal history, narratives and storytelling. Within this approach, Park believes learning goes beyond data analysis to sharing, speaking and exchanging actions against the background of common experience, tradition, history and culture (Park, 1993). The fieldwork mainly consists of informal dialogue with people within their own circumstances and environments. These discussions have taken place in shops (Berridge Road), in Mosques (Karimia), at weddings (conference centre) and funerals (Islamic Centre St. Anns.) There are also more formal interviews that the author has conducted with stakeholders, community activists and a sample of participants. These interviews are open-ended and have been recorded over a period of time.

This way the study explores the ways through which various power-sensitive perspectives, emerging from a number of conflicting realities and multiplicities, operate and constitute subjectivities. For such an understanding, power needs to be seen as relational and dynamic, and not something that is absolute and static. This way the thesis works with the circulatory model of power, something which is not attached to the structures, but circulates continuously in social relations. This conceptualization sees power not just repressive and constraining but productive and enabling wherein individuals 'simultaneously undergo and exercise power' (Foucault, 1980).

The discourse of social exclusion, which is the combination of many social, cultural and economic conditions, is impossible to explore from a monolithic standpoint. This analysis demands a framework that recognizes social exclusion as a discourse of various relationships, positions and situations. Within such a framework, one perspective one tool to fit all is not tenable. Arguments against using a multi-perspective and multi-disciplinary approach mostly emanate from the positivist research tradition which sees life and experience as neat concepts which can be easily put into compartments. This compartmentalization of human experiences cannot explain the 'messiness' of existence. Rather than viewing research as a series of hermetic stages, modern methodology conceives research as process:

> *It does not follow a neat pattern but is a messy interaction between the research problem, the design of the research and data collection and analysis.* (Brewer, 2000: 102)

One of the criticism of this methodology is an inherent conflict between three theoretical perspectives: feminism, poststructuralism and liberation theology, used to develop this framework. There are common apprehensions and shared interest that bring these perspectives closer to offer epistemological plurality needed to maps out possibilities. This process is facilitated by adopting a non- conventional framework, and learning from various disciplines, including cultural studies, sociology, theology and human geography. The study accepts the fact that these disciplines and approaches are not mutually exclusive but overlap and inter-weave as happens in real life. We also need to walk away from the monolithic conception of feminism as a singular body of knowledge to understand patriarchy or a single action to correct the injustices and inequalities. Many feminists, especially the post-modern and black feminists, argue that there is no concrete "womens' experience" from which to construct knowledge, and that the diversity of womens' experiences cannot be generalised (Narayan, 1989; Benhabib, 1995). Similarly, liberation theology is not one single way of relating social aspects of life with the spiritual. The liberation theology as practised in Latin America is different from that practised in North America, which is again different from Europe. While the ordained priesthood and parts of the Roman Catholic Church remain opposed to liberation theology, at the grassroots many practitioners are making spirituality relevant to the lives of marginalized people. Liberation theology, however, is fragmented in the way it is practised by feminist theologians, black theologians and so on.

These multiple meanings and understandings of feminism, poststructuralism, and liberation theology offer enough space to look at the common concerns and interests within these positions to develop shared strategies. Thus the methodology, the author is developing for this study is actually this productive 'coming together' of these apparently differing perspectives. But this is not a synthetic process but a creative way of looking at things differently. The study does not claim to create the body of knowledge by using this framework but, as has been mentioned before, a way of looking at issues differently within a range possibilities.

Weedon (1997) maintains that the least 'a feminist poststructuralism can do is explain the assumptions underlying the questions asked and answered by other forms of feminist theory, making their political assumptions explicit' (1997:20). The framework draws support from this intersection of feminism and poststructuralism to address questions about social power and relations are structured around gender, class and race. Weedon says that the historical perspective present in Michel Foucault's work is very relevant in such analysis (ibid). One of the key preoccupations of feminism is gender relations which cannot be seen in isolation from other social relations and power like racism, homophobia, disability and ageism. This research project is not a feminist project in the sense that it exclusively looks at gender, but the marginalisation of women is a contributory factor that helps to understand other injustices and inequalities. One more risk in this approach is the possibility of a 'pick and choose' approach and an over-emphasis on qualitative methods, which in turn can lead to over- enthusiasm – a new 'orthodoxy' to replace an existing orthodoxy. Choosing one method or methodological approach to deal with complex social and cultural issues is untenable with this research project, partly due to the fact that the thesis is rooted in an epistemology that claims there are various possibilities in knowing and living. Secondly, the study walks away from the positivist approach and rejects the socio-scientific concept of one problem, one method, one solution, as no one method and methodological approach can be always correct in all situations. Looking at various tools available to gather and analyze the field information, PAR may have some technical lacunae, but its advantage in experiencing and validation is worth the risk rather than adopting a technically sound positivist and essentialist method rooted in quantitative research, which is diametrically opposite to the objectives and goals of this study.

It has been argued earlier that the objectives and context of this study demand a more emancipatory methodology where 'conscious subjectivity' is favoured over 'assumed objectivity' and where theory and practice operate within the same discursive space. The author draw support from the critical feminist methodologies which prefer 'conscious partiality' over 'detached objectivity'. This is vital in the study of marginalised groups who are voiceless. But this approach poses not only the methodological problems but also ethical issues like 'using and abusing' the trust and the possible harm the publication of research findings can cause to those researched.

By making his research objectives explicit, the fieldwork is drawn from day to day living experiences, and the author does not divorce his living experiences from those he tries to explore. Raghuram et al. (1998), identifying emancipatory goals and stressing awareness about ethics and self-reflexivity of feminist methodologies, provide a justification for this validation. Secondly, the Freirian principle of conscientization lends support to actions that enhance the critical consciousness of the oppressed; a framework that is dialectical and engages with oppressive social structures (Harvey, 1990). However, author's position and the political agenda for this research could incline the author towards over-enthusiasm and simplification. The author has explicated his situation, and how he negotiates way through the moral, ethical and professional maze this study presents. The author writes the study thesis in the first person. This helps the reader to easily locate him within the text. This is both a methodological and epistemological requirement of this work because the author's position and the way he observes the field is crucial to understanding this work. Writing in the first person also removes the doubts about the objectivity in fieldwork.

The study is rooted in author's deep commitment to empowerment of the powerless, and shares the epistemological position that the world we live in is shaped by the relations of power and that the only way to make change is to change the equilibrium of these relations. Developing an organic framework, which brings together emancipatory perspectives and applying it through Participatory Action Research is the closest we can get to challenge hegemony and create 'chaos in authority' and acknowledge other worldviews (Gramsci, 1971).

The study is an insider's account of how people reflect on situations, debate issues and engage in actions, and being there and being part of this whole process adds to the subjective account the study intends to offer. This familiarity implies a greater intimacy with people and their lives but also has a greater chance of manipulation and misuse. Stacey (1988) argues that ethnographic methods could expose the researched to a greater risk of exploitation and betrayal than through positivist research. The author keeps on questioning his research objectives, his motives and reasons for being in the middle of all this. This questioning is quite taxing to the author's work, and me, and on many occasions the questioning leads to self-doubt. But every bout of questioning is followed by reflections, which helps me to change, transform and adapt in the process of reacting to these questions. Overall, the author's belief in seeing knowledge and experience through a multitude of possibilities and a commitment to validation of other ways of living keeps me going through various stages of questioning and reasoning.

Participatory action research (PAR) seeks empowerment of subjects by incorporating them in the identification of problems, information-gathering and analysis. Other methods and methodologies, in contrast, keep the researched at distance from the researcher. So by not giving the subjects the opportunity to explore, collect, evaluate and decide, such methods reinforce orthodoxies. As an action research project, this study, however, is in the hands of the subjects of this work. The author sees his role more as a facilitator to enable radio broadcasting as a platform for discussion, reflection and action. Traditionally academicians are seen as outsiders, living in ivory towers- far from the living experiences of people. In academy, activists are seen as enthusiasts who try to over-simplify complex situations and issues. Being in this situation, the author finds these concerns stemming from the tendency to separate theory from practice. In his role as community worker and in his responsibility as an academician, the author constantly tries to overcome the researcher – researched divide, and let theory learn from practice and vice versa.

Notes

1. The Radio Authority (now OfCom) in the UK would allow community and special interest groups to broadcast on FM and AM for a limited period of time to celebrate festivals and events. This limited licensing would be normally for a period of one month and was called Restricted Service License or RSL. The Radio Authority was responsible for licensing and regulating Independent Radio in accordance with the statutory requirements of the Broadcasting Acts 1990 and 1996. It plans frequencies, awards licences, regulates programming and advertising, and plays an active role in the discussion and formulation of policies which affect the Independent Radio industry and its listeners.

Chapter 4
Discursive Space

Although political mobilization of ethnic minorities in the UK is well documented, most of the debate has remained confined around race relations. The brand of cultural pluralism promoted by British Race Relations –on the principle of racial equality- has come under severe criticism for failing to understand the complexity of race and ignoring the spatio-temporal realities in which marginalized groups live. Diversity, difference, religion and ethnic origin have become important seats of contestation and consensus within minorities. But this theorisation has been criticised for 'legitimising inequality' and leading to rejection of those cultures which do not correspond to the nation state (Samad, 2004).

At a time when demands for equality and opportunity are not only made within broader racial categories, but within religious orientation, ethnic origin and nationality (Paul Statham, 1999), one can see the erosion in multiculturalism, which bundled all non-white categories together for political and administrative correctness.

Whether we agree with the relevance of multiculturalism or not, we cannot deny the fact that ethnic/minority/racial assertiveness is not just a demand for equal opportunity on the basis of ethnicity, colour, race but faith, tradition and identity are becoming part of a new emphasis by 'others' who demand respect for otherness. This renewed assertiveness is not exclusive to ethnic or minority politics alone, but many more areas including sexuality and feminism, have been arguing for long that 'equality is not enough'. Demanding emancipation and the transformation of society, these movements want liberation from existing frameworks, values and systems.

As envisioned in the previous chapter, the study takes a non- essential and multi-perspective approach in learning from the experiences, which may be local and specific to a context, but can also become apparent across ethnicities, geographies and identities. So, both epistemologically and methodologically, unpacking the concept of community is critical to this study, which engaging with the worldviews of the Muslim population of South Asian origin living in inner city Nottingham. These worldviews, expressed and validated through a community based radio station, reveal many commonalities and contradictions within the concept of community,

F. Malik, *Addressing Health Inequalities through Community Media*,
https://doi.org/10.1007/978-3-031-35237-9_4

especially when seen within complex spatial and historical contexts. The study acknowledging the diversity and dynamisms within the concept, theorizes it as a discursive space where similarities and differences are negotiated for 'expanded consciousness' (Freire, 1972) essential to 'democratic participation and empowerment.

This study is about the worldviews of the people of South Asian origin (*Mirpuri community*/Pakistani), living in inner city Nottingham (Radford, Hyson Green, Forest Fields, Sneinton), sharing locally the social, economic and political aspects of being a 'immigrant, Muslim, coloured, disadvantaged' minority. Both epistemologically and methodologically, the concept of community is central to this study as it acknowledges the heterogeneities and diversities embedded and performed within this community. It is as much about differences as it is about similarity and identity (Gilroy, 1982).

Historically reliance and dependency on kinship, which many immigrant communities of south Asian origin illustrate, has led many first generation immigrants to live in the same area, even on the same street. This living in a pattern of 'home communities' as 'concentration from particular villages leads to 'clustering of people' as a tendency to 'gravitate towards shared culture' (Anwar, 1979; Desai, 1963). Many scholars, though, contest the concept of community and identity, raising the question about the 'legitimacy of such constructs as Pakistani community'. These scholars emphasize that the notion of the community can 'suppress difference' and highlight the lack of homogeneity and presence of multiple identities within what is perceived from outside and often experienced from within a single community (Young, 1990a, b; Eade, 1989; Shaw, 1988). Iris Young (1990a, b), while stressing the need to acknowledge 'difference', argues for a differentiated citizenship and group representation instead of a conception that suppresses difference. Solmos and Back (1995) have cast doubt on the unproblematic use of the notion of community, culture and identity. Amit and Rapport (2002) argue that with the dislocation of the conventional connection between individuals and collectives in a global system of production, labour, law and political identity in which political, economic and cultural connections are ever increasing, the very ontology of community as a mobilised social group is uncertain.

Despite uncertainties, the concept of community continues to remain a basis for 'collective class action' (Castells, 1983), 'a source of identity, of moral and social stability', (Revill, 1993), 'difference and unity' (Day & Murdoch, 1993), both in terms of 'aspiration and principle' (Warburton, 1998) and a 'place of amity, mutual support, and homeliness' (Bauman, 2000). Community is also seen as 'strategic, situational and fluid' (Massey, 1991; Laclau, 1994). Alongside these positive descriptions, the concept is also seen to justify exercising social control, restraining dissent (Taylor, 1997), and used as a site for social engineering (Forrest & Kearns, 1999). These descriptions, explanations and application of the concept show a variety of analyses and help to reflect on the ambiguity and ambivalence the concept entails.

Community is not just the communal union of people. It is also about common perceptions about social justice and myriad the connections between people within a group. The Gemeinschaft shallow understanding of community has come under criticism for failing to realize the inner dynamism with the concept of community. However, the 'politics of difference' helps to understand the concept of community in new ways. There is, however, a risk of imagining and perpetuating labels based on prejudice, ignorance and sheer generalisations. The literature on the subject shows that there is a tendency to construct and disseminate inaccurate labels about people (Hall, 1997), particularly about sub groups within communities. The unproblematic creation of the notion of the Pakistani community is one example of this generalisation, which often ignores the diversity within these groups in terms of class, religion, gender, caste as well as the range of geographical and historical contingencies (Brah, 1996). The diversity within Muslim populations, as well as among the South Asians and what is constructed as the Pakistani community, has repeatedly been emphasised in ethnographic studies (Shaw, 1988; Modood et al., 1997).

So, how does the author deal with this paradox, especially when the author's arguments draw support from critical, poststructuralist and feminist perspectives, which reject generalisations, uniformities and universalities? There is no single definition of community which can encompass everything a community can or cannot achieve. Neither is there a universal explanation of this concept that can fit in all situations at all times. However, this does not negate the possibility of people sharing certain aspects of culture and experience as they face similar sets of problems (racism, discrimination and cultural disadvantage). Differences are part of human life, and living together means accepting difference and finding ways of working with them. Such an association expresses the members' commitment to the continuity and perpetuation of the group (Werbner, 2005).

On the other hand, a complex discourse of being non-white, represented as culturally different (Hall, 1997) and being from former British colonies (Barrera, 1979:194) create multiple disadvantages for the immigrant communities within the unfavourable deprived urban areas where they are concentrated. This discourse creates a culture of exclusion, which is further aggravated by the barriers to access and participation (Hardill et al., 2001). As a result of this exclusion, people gravitate towards a community which provides both a refuge and means to contest exclusion. Jeffery (1976:182) highlights this attraction towards a collectivity as a 'conscious re-assertion of Pakistani-ness'. As in the case of other groups and communities, there is no doubt about the diversity within the South Asian Diaspora, but there are also striking similarities within these groups, particularly in the patterns of immigration and settlement between various Asian communities in the UK.

Avtar Brah chronicles the various stages of the settlement of Asian community in Post war Britain as; 'coming to Vilayat' (1950s to 1960s), 'a home away from home' (1960s to 1970s) and 'here to stay' (1970s to 1980s). The Mirpuri/ Pakistani community's chain migration, which has allowed village and kin networks to be reproduced in the UK, is well documented (Anwar, 1979; Dayha, 1974). The kin network in the form of Biradari facilitates living in extended and joint families in proximity to each other. In sociological terms ethnic groups are understood to share the belief in their common origin and heritage. Bacal (1991) relates this shared belief to historical memories of colonisation and migration. These experiences, Bacal stresses, are essential for the 'propagation of the group'. On the basis of common origin and similar experience, ethnic groups have been distinguished from others in cultural terms like language, religion, tribe, nationality and race (Stavenhagen, 1986). Members of this group share some 'phenotypic, cultural, linguistic, religious, national features or combination of some of these or all of these factors' (Bacal, 1991:80).

Alongside these internal dynamics, a range of outside influences also pull these people together, although this coming together is not permanent and never complete. The official, political, media and academic discourses group non-white groups together in various categories ranging from Black to immigrant to disadvantaged to faith-based, for their own convenience and purpose. The discourse of social exclusion is seen to reduce people to labels and numbers without looking into the contextual and structural issues, which disempower people. When mixed with other racial categories like Asian, Black, coloured, non-white, the process not only stigmatises the marginality but also puts the blame of exclusion on the victims of exclusion. It is not just the racism but a populist discourse based on tabloid press and street politics that gives credence to these labels, and eventually brings them into the administrative processes. Often in literature and policy documents, it is seen that the membership of the ethnic minority and various forms of disadvantage like dependence on social benefits, lifestyle led health issues, higher rates of unemployment, poor levels of participation, forced marriages, parallel lives, etc., are used interchangeably to give the impression of a problematic underclass.

Although the race and poverty is more abundant in literature, many authors see it ideological rather than empirical. Paul Spicker (2002) emphatically argues that poverty is an economic risk that can affect everyone and not a moral or social problem. This process of 'othering', is seen to be the result of racism and discrimination and even ignorance. This process is understood leading to a 'refused identity and identification within the majority nation, having to find some other roots on which to stand on' (Hall, 1991:52). The media feed on this categorization and perpetuate it further, giving a public legitimacy to this terminology. The state machinery in the shape of public services promote these images further. Saeeda Shah (1998) argues these images come from the situated dealings and interaction of public services like heath, education and social services:

> *Across ambiguities, misunderstandings and misconceptions, images are constructed which highlight the differences and increase distances. The atmosphere of uncertainty, coupled with exclusion, leads to the encapsulation of immigrant groups, and subsequently develops and strengthens the sense of group belongingness round a concept of community which can be at times politically useful and psychologically satisfying.* (Shah, 1998: 51)

The thesis acknowledges the slipperiness of the concept of the community, but it does not accept the explanation of extreme individualisation, complete breakdown of relationships and irrelevance of identity on the basis that we live in a globalised, post-modern times. The author believes that with the growing insecurities of the present times and fears about the future, there is a renewed interest in collectiveness, which is deliberate and considered. The growing influence of civil society, global anti-capitalist movements, anti-war lobbies and more specifically, the increasing influence of Islamic revivalist movements based on an Ummatic concept of unity within Muslims, illustrates the fact that globalisation does not only break affiliations but in certain cases facilitates new associations.

These new associations might not be a self-sustaining village communities but more interdependent widely scattered groups who share a common interest. At the same time, at a very local level, people discover ways and means to find strength in communal relationship when their identity. With the significance of faith-based institutions growing and a desire to use these institutions to complement social and cultural development, more young people are getting attracted toward identity politics. In the case of the Muslim community, especially the Mirpuri community, the institution of the mosque adds more value to this collectivity. While for the elderly people it remains the focus of their worship, the younger generations find it a dynamic social space as well.

Muslims of South Asian origin constitute almost three quarters of the adherents of Islam in Britain (ONS, UK). The census of 2001 showed the largest number of Muslims in Britain originates from Pakistan (687,592) followed by Bangladesh (261,833) and India (133,783). There are also sizeable groups from the Middle East, North Africa, the Far East and Eastern Europe. Though the theory of Orientalism has universal applications, it can be best understood in the contexts of former colonies. Colonialism, which marked the start of the decline of the Muslim empire in many parts of the world, had a huge influence on the Muslim psyche. This decline leads to a process of Islamic revivals and reform. This process, in turn, gave birth to a number of variations in Islam (Francis Robinson, 1988). Over a period of time, as the immigrants from South Asia became more settled in Britain, Islamic movements of South Asia also became visible here. Francis Robinson (1988: 2) writes that these different movements, ways of being Muslim and the relationships between these movements is often 'abrasive'. He writes that the origins and orientations of the groups are important in understanding their behaviour in British society.

Concept of Community in Islam

In another article, Raghuram (1999) envisions the revival of religion as an expression of socio-cultural particularism against the universalising tendencies of globalization, though she thinks this distinction is unstable. While the community shares one faith, their responses to issues are local, temporal and strategic. The contemporary tensions between many Islamic societies and the West' are seen by many scholars as the result of historical processes.

The word *Ummah* occurs 64 times in the Quran, underlining its importance in social and political conduct. The standard understanding of the word is 'community' and its root word in Arabic language is 'umm', which means mother (Al-Ahsan, 1992). In Quran (2/143), Ummah or community or nation of Islam is described as the 'median' among the peoples and nations implying stability and harmony. However, there are a number of interpretations of this description ranging from political and ideological influence (Al-Faruqi, 1982) to more of a spiritual and social force (Khan, 1997).

The Prophet Muhammad (PBUH), who established the first community of Muslims in Medina after he fled the persecution in Makkah, stresses the importance of Community. According to *Hadith* (saying of Prophet), narrated by *Al Bukhari*[1] (vol. I, 291), the Prophet said: 'the Muslim community is like a body if one part hurts, the whole body feels the pain.'

On the basis of the importance given to the concept of community in Islam, aspiration to live as a community is stronger among Muslims. Islam is followed in many parts of the world, and Muslims tend to live in communities giving local colours and flavours to a universal message. It is important to emphasise that the message of Islam no doubt is universal, but it does not prescribe a monolithic universal community to practice this message.

[13]Sahih al_bukari, as it is commonly known, is one of the six canonical Prophetic traditions *(Hadith)*. These were collected by the Muslim scholar, Muhammad ibn Ismail al-Bukhari (810–870) and complied during his life time. Most Sunni Muslim view this as a the most trusted collection of *Hadith* and the authentic source after the Qur'an.

Islam does not believe in a homogenous and undifferentiated community but encourages diversity. Contrary to the common belief that the Muslim community is a universal concept that does not take into account regional and local variations, the Quran emphasises unity in diversity:

> *O' mankind! We created you from a single (pair) of a male and female, and made you into Nations and tribes, that may know each other. Verily the most honoured of you in the sight of Allah is (he who is) the most righteous of you.* (Quran, 49:13)

However, a hermeneutic approach to religion is disputed by many sociologists. In his influential social analysis of religion, Bryan S Turner (1993) argues that such an approach focuses too much on social action ignoring social structures that can shape action. Turner argues that the religion serves as an institutional link between economic and human reproduction. He further writes that reformist philosophy of Islam supported rational civilization, modern capitalism and democracy.

Muslims of South Asian origin constitute almost three quarters of the adherents of Islam in Britain (ONS, UK). The census of 2001 shows the largest number of Muslims in Britain originates from Pakistan (687,592) followed by Bangladesh (261,833) and India (133,783). There are also sizeable groups from the Middle East, North Africa, the Far East and Eastern Europe.

After influencing social and political life in South Asia, many Islamic movements Islam have spread to other parts of the world. The contemporary Muslim society in the UK, which mostly comprises of South Asian Muslims, exhibits Barailvi, Davebandi, Wahabbi, Tablegi Jamat and Jamat Islami movements in more defined way (Robinson, 1988). These groups push their interpretations and range from very purinitcal to a Sufi shades of Islam. This way, the concept of a monolith community looks far-fetched. Another problem with the idea of community is the choices and preferences of identities and labels used in describing people from various countries and origins.

These preferences/labels have pan- Islamic, nationalistic, localised, and at times linguistic and cultural overtones. We often hear labels and proclamations like 'Iranian revolutionary; or 'Indonesian nationalist; or 'Arab socialist' or 'Turkish Liberal' or 'Pakistani fundamentalist' or 'Indian Sufi', 'rich sheikhs' or 'Palestinian fighters', Afghan Mujahedeen, 'Kashmiri fighters' and so on. This plurality, often forced from outside and at times proclaimed internally, dilutes the 'purity' of an imagined Islamic identity which seeks a seamless *Ummatic* community.

Adhering to a puritan Islamic identity risks alienation from the mainstream, which can lead to exclusion and separatism? This is the predicament many Muslim communities face. There are obvious tensions between imagining an ideal puritan and 'seamless *Ummah*' and living in a fragmented and profane world. The responses to this dilemma are varied and, at times, confusing. Abdurrahman Wahid says:

> *The challenge at this time is to find an identity that will both develop a sense of belonging to Islam while also retaining a sense of belonging to a larger and wider network of groups motivated by world ideologies, other faiths, and global concerns.* (Wahid, 2001: 55)

This modernising agenda is lost in the 'publicly orchestrated confrontation' with the West and Western values through which younger generations are lured into an ideology' to create a 'political version of *Ummah*' (Khan, 1997). While at the global level these new politically motivated identities are manifesting in different forms of protest against their own governments and regimes in the Western countries with sizable Muslim minorities, there seems to be a generational shift in identity among the young who are finding Britishness and being Muslim less conflicting. In this shift, Muslims 'retain some notions of community' to justify their antagonistic stance against the police and white gangs, whose 'modes of violence tend to be individualistic' (Samad, 2004:22).

Looking at the Muslim population in the UK, it is younger and mostly concentrated in the poor neighbourhoods in inner city areas. This concentration of Muslim communities in urban post-industrial cities adds one more dimension to the concept of community. Living in proximity and sharing a faith, along with 'back-home' family connections and an alienation from the mainstream society, forges a sense of closeness, which is then reflected as identity. This is close to three definitions of community: a geographical locality, a local social system and a sense of identity (Newby, 1980:3). In theory, community ultimately embraces all the believers, regardless of their gender, colour, nationality or any other such variation. Strong emphasis is placed on family, kinship, and neighbours. In order to feel secure, religion is used like a shield. Certain aspects of the pivotal teachings of Islam receive particular emphasis in the interplay with regional subcultures. In the South Asian community Islamic teaching and injunctions regarding immediate and extended family and neighbours and other Muslims are reinforced by the local patterns of behaviour concerning the family and the Biradari (clan/tribe).

These real and imagined factors of physical and psychological proximities have strengthened communal bonds of togetherness which Anwar thinks lead to 'encapsulation' (Anwar, 1979). Desai makes the observation that the clustering of immigrants in streets of some areas points to the tendency to gravitate towards shared culture (Desai, 1963:22). Stuart Hall argues strongly that the formulation of an ethnic identity is 'essentially a politically and culturally constructed category' (Hall, 1992a, b, p. 259), and draws attention to the 'issues of representation' and 'ambivalence of identification and desire in his discussion of new ethnicities' (1992a, b: 255).

The group identity becomes more assertive during the fasting month of Ramadan when Radio Ramzan complements the celebration of faith (the ritual of fasting). In a local situation, the radio helps to forge that communal feeling by organizing communal activities and serving as a community-wide loudspeaker to inform and engage in debates and discussions that touch the lives of Muslims. Radio Ramzan has grown within a variety of other Muslim media, side by side with the political mobilisation and cultural assertiveness among the minority ethnic groups. Establishing its own media has been part of the strategy to counter Islamophobia (Runnymede Trust, 1997) and present a more balanced point of view. These media have also provided new social spaces for young Muslims.

The Muslim population in Britain is very diverse. The people of Pakistani descent make up the largest group of Muslims in the UK, of which about two thirds are from the Mirpur and Kotli district of 'Pakistan Administered Kashmir', who are increasing rapidly in size, 'because of fertility rate' and as a result of ongoing 'processes of family reunion' (Ballard, 2002). There are almost 400,000 Mirpuris living in the U.K, While Kashmir is a very strong influence in the way the Mirpuri community project and represent them, it is also Muslim and 'Pakistani identity' which describes this community. Stuart Hall argues that the formulation of an ethnic identity' is essentially a politically and culturally constructed category; and draws attention to the 'issues of representation' and 'ambivalence of identification and desire' (Hall, 1997). Mirpuri/ Kashmiri/ Pakistani identity which many of these people prefer is part of this uncertainty about Kashmir and their strong emotional links with the dispute. They call themselves differently in different situations. Mirpuri identity is linguistic and cultural, Kashmiri identity is emotional and aspirational, and Pakistani identity is practical, while the Muslim identity encompasses all these identities.

The *Karimia Mosque* at the heart of the community in Forest Fields in Nottingham opened up the possibility for young people to get involved in sports, recreation activities, and homework clubs in a faith-based environment, which mainstream activities cannot provide. Besides, being a place for worship, it has pool tables, table tennis facilities, computers, and also organises trips and sports. A charity named 'Muslim Hands' was also started from the premises of this mosque. This charity is now one of the largest Muslim charities in the UK, raising around four million pounds every years and it employs about 15 local young people (Muslim Hands, 2001). But this is just one mosque normally used by the *Barailve* followers of Islam. There are other mosques and institutions in Nottingham offering a wide range of activities, and are popular among their followers.

To theorise ethnic/racial inequality, let's take a look at various concepts put forward to understand this phenomenon from social, economic and cultural standpoints. The deficiency theory sees 'backwardness', inferior intelligence and low moral attribute (Jenson, 1969, 1973). The socio-cultural deficiency approach blames deficiencies in social and cultural organisation (Lewis, 1959). It is argued that the sources of inequality lie in the prejudice, discrimination and racial ideologies practiced by majority groups (Barrera, 1979), and the social-structural theories believe the division is on the basis of class, race, ethnicity and gender and the privileged position of dominant groups (Cox, 1948/1970). Racism in different forms and guises has been recognized as a major prejudice against the people of non-white colour. But when such prejudice becomes part of official and political discourse, it discriminates against and marginalizes people. In 1999, institutional racism was acknowledged to be present within organizations and institutions of British society. Sir William McPherson in the report, The Stephen Lawrence Inquiry (1999) defined institutional racism as:

> *The collective failure of an organization to provide an appropriate and professional service to people because of their colour, culture or ethnic origin. It can be seen or detected in processes, attitudes and behaviour which amount to discrimination through unwitting prejudice, ignorance, thoughtlessness and racist stereotyping which disadvantages minority ethnic people.* (Macpherson report, 1999)

Many scholars identify the legacy of colonialism and the growing influence of capitalism as a reason for sustained racism in British society (Wallerstein, 1974; Bacal, 1991). The colonial legacy and its mindset are believed to be playing a big part in the way immigrant communities are understood and treated in the Western democracies. With more and more people from former colonies coming to the UK for work and family reasons, an 'internal colonialism' is seen to be defining 'geographies of the metropolis' (Barrera, 1979). On similar lines, Bacal, (1991) argues that the colonial heritage is responsible for complicating the class with race and ethnicity within the colony and the colonial metropolis. He writes: This ascriptive process as a relative social condition implies a psychological pressure experienced by ethnic group members, to define themselves with ethnic attributes, namely, in terms of an 'ethnic identity' (Bacal, 1991: 66). Whatever the claims and theoretical explanation, ethnic identities in various multi-cultural societies have not vanished. There is, in fact, a resurgence of ethnic and racial identities, and minorities are becoming more conscious of their rights and position in multi-cultural societies. Minority cultures and identities have survived both the forces of modernisation and the coercion of totalitarianism. But that does not mean that structural imbalances are not there anymore. Social inequality, racism and discrimination continue to suppress the subordinate ethnic groups (McPherson, 1999).

There is no clear link between poverty and race, but the available data confirms that some groups experience a more disproportionate disadvantage and social exclusion than others. However, the minority ethnic communities are more likely to experience poverty, unemployment, lower educational qualifications, suffer ill health, and live in poorer quality housing. Furthermore, they may also be subject to racial harassment and racist crime (SEU, 2000). Employment is generally lower for all minority ethnic groups, and the lowest rates are found among Pakistanis and Bangladeshis. Women's employment rates are far lower than men with only 28 percent of Pakistani women and 23 per cent of Bangladeshi women economically active, compared with 73 percent of Pakistani men and 69 percent of Bangladeshi men. The proportion of self-employment among Muslim groups is diverse with it being relatively high for Pakistanis at 22 percent and around 13 percent and 12 percent for Indians and Bangladeshi, which is near the rates found for White British 11 percent (Annual Local Area Labour Force Survey, 2001/02). Similarly, in England, members of particular black and minority ethnic groups, particular the Pakistani, Bangladeshi and African-Caribbean groups suffer the poorest health (Nazroo, 1997). Scholars argue that greater emphasis on ethnic identity and culture, racial discrimination, and people's participation are important factors in removing health inequalities (Nazroo, 1998; Williams et al., 1997). The Race/discrimination/exclusion is the most important discourse within the meta-discourse of multiculturalism that affects minorities in the UK. Although these perspectives are not similar, the reason to keep them together is the inescapable interrelation and interdependence of this experience.

Social inequality is not the only issue that affects the day to day living of minority groups. The fixed and situated categorisation of these groups by academia and media creates and reinforces discourses in which and through which difference is demonised. These people are seen and stereotyped on the basis of situated categories and associations, which emerge from the vicious circle of media, academia and politics. Consequently, labels and myths of fundamentalism, terrorism, domestic violence, illegal immigration, troubles in the Middle East are associated with the Muslim community. However, the group consciousness among the immigrants varies from generation to generation. While the first generation South Asians shared a deep rooted homeland consciousness which defined their individual and collective social, cultural and political life in Britain, for the second and third generation born and brought up here, the consciousness is more a result of the struggle between personal identity which they develop in wider society (especially in schools) and that which they acquire at home (dominated by parents). Modood et al. (1994:59) see this struggle culminating in 'ethnic pride', which comes from the affirmation of roots and impressions from the contemporary society, which looks down at their 'ethnicity with inferiority'. He adds that religion is considered a 'distinctive heritage and ethnic identity' of this consciousness.

Highlighting this changing nature of a group, Michael Banton says that groups, whether based on ethnicity, nationality, religion or race, are always changing in a 'triangular web of structure, process and consciousness' (Banton, 1997:117). Michael Banton (1997) emphasises that it is the collective action and purpose of individuals in a group that fosters the sense of community. Quoting Max Weber's description of associational and communal collective action, Banton (1997: 117) argues that 'an association of persons sharing common ethnic origin would appeal to a consciousness of shared experience and would therefore be communal from the outset' as group support and collective action becomes indispensable for such consciousness. British Muslims have exhibited overt political mobilisation on many issues by uniting tactically despite differences, and forming wider coalitions with socialists, Christians, anti-war activists, liberals, as a strategy to show their displeasure with government policy on Afghanistan and Iraq. Though this dissatisfaction, which relates directly to religion and ethnicity, it rarely conflicted with Muslims Britishness and their belonging to British society.

These arguments illustrate the strategic and tactical positioning of the community to deal with both internal and external dynamics. This re-conceptualisation of community is also fuelled by the change from essentialised 'Black politics' to a wider perspective where political and social mobilisation of different ethnic groups is privileged (Hall, 1988; Solmos & Back, 1995). Writing about the 'embodied' nature of social and cultural rituals of South Asian migrants, Werbner (2005) argues that such representation are 'substantiated in objects, food and substances that inscribe and transform the person and constitute his or her felt subjectivity'. In her study of the Pakistani-Asian community in the UK, she finds the religious rituals, cultural practices, and social events becoming a 'mode of transaction, relatedness and embodiment' (2005:11–12). At the local level, however, such politics takes a different turn when local power struggles, competition for resources, and fragmented identities become more important than national alliances and international solidarities. Here, broader categories start breaking into smaller and more specific identities and definitions.

This observation lends support to the author's conceptualisation of the Mirpuri community in which he finds political and cultural identities around race and ethnicity in a flux. Categories of religion, minoritism, race, locality, and gender are included and excluded as part of a strategy to position itself differently in different situations and under different circumstances. This strategic approach thus helps to engage with myriad power relations which characterize community politics. In line with these arguments, the thesis understands community as a dynamic discursive space where power relations, commonalties and diversities keep on changing situationally and strategically.

Note

1. Sahih al_bukari, as it is commonly known, is one of the six canonical Prophetic traditions (Hadith). These were collected by the Muslim scholar, Muhammad ibn Ismail al-Bukhari (810–870) and complied during his life time. Most Sunni Muslim view this as a the most trusted collection of Hadith and the authentic source after the Qur'an.

Chapter 5
Beyond Healthism

The enjoyment of the highest attainable standard of health is one of the fundamental rights of every human being without distinction of race, religion, political belief, economic or social condition (World Health Organization)

As the Covid-19 pandemic spread across the globe, it interacted with prevailing inequalities and widened the gulf between the health outcomes of the privileged groups and those socially and economically disadvantaged. Covid affected people's health, resulted in deaths and nearly collapsed the health services even in many parts of the developing world. However, the extent of damage has been significantly higher in areas where the disadvantaged people, most racial and ethnic groups live, under deprived conditions. The impact of this pandemic on communities living in poor neighbourhoods, with low-income populations and minority ethnic groups has been very disproportionate, uncovering appalling inequalities that exist, and are on increase, across the world. Be it the spread of Covid-19 infection, hospitalization, symptom severity, need for critical care, long Covid and deaths, poor, vulnerable, Black and Minority Ethnic people and low wage workers have suffered unequally. More evidence of the disproportionate effect of Covid-19 is emerging from the underlying socio, economic, contextual, geographical and racial issues that underline a direct link between social disadvantage and poor health outcomes.

Drawing on historical data of the Spanish Flue of 1908 and the H1N1 outbreak of 2019, Bambra et al. (2021), highlight the continuity in health inequalities that exist in many parts of the developed world. Despite the progress made in scientific breakthroughs, socio-economic factors along with the discrimination disadvantaged people face making even the most developed countries most unequal when it comes to health and wellbeing. Bambra et al. (2021) citing Covid-19 data from some of the poor neighbourhoods in Spain, the US, Canada, Sweden and the UK, explain how the rate of infection, need for critical care, the prevalence of effects of long Covid and mortality rates due to pandemic have been much higher in poor neighbourhoods of Barcelona, Illinois, Toronto, Stockholm and deprived inner-city areas in North East England.

F. Malik, *Addressing Health Inequalities through Community Media*,
https://doi.org/10.1007/978-3-031-35237-9_5

There is a general understanding among the policymakers, academics and medical professionals that the Covid-19 had a disproportionate effect on ethnic minority groups in the UK. Pre and post-pandemic evidence collected from various inner-city areas with a higher proportion of minority ethnic people support the argument that disadvantaged people were disproportionately affected by the Covid 19 (Ocloo, 2021; Bambra et al. 2021). In the UK, initial research illustrated that the people living in deprived communities had double the diagnosis rates of the pandemic for both men and women. Similarly, lower socioeconomic groups exhibited higher rates of long term impacts like neurological and respiratory symptoms along with fatigue which needed longer hospital stays. As per the Public Health England, during the early phase of the pandemic, the first quarter of 2020, were more than double in 20% of most-deprived neighbourhoods. Similar disparities were observed in death rates in different regions. As per Public Health England, 57.7 more people/100,000 died due to Covid in the Northern region than in the rest of England (Bambra et al., 2021). Health inequalities were also observed in terms of peoples' occupations. According to the Office of National Statistics (220 a), in England and Wales, death rates in the early stages of the Covid pandemic (March to May 2020) were seen among people who worked as construction workers, security guards, cleaners, nurses, care workers, ambulance drivers, administrative and secretarial workers while the mortality due to this Covid was lowest among managers, directors, senior and professional workers.

Black, Asian and Minority Ethnic Communities (BAME) exhibited stark inequalities as a result of the Covid 19 pandemic in the UK. Public Health England (2020), noticed that BAME populations showed a higher death risk than the White British population with Black British and Bangladeshi British populations having twice the death risk, and the risk of death increased by 10% and 50% across the Indian, Pakistani, Chinese, Caribbean and Other Black ethnic groups. The higher rates of mortality due to the COVID-19 pandemic among the Black and Minority Ethnic groups in the UK once again reveal health inequalities that exist on account of socio-economic disadvantage, morbidity due to diabetes, coronary diseases and obesity on one hand and the experiences of racism, discrimination and fear on the other. The Public Health England report to ascertain the impact of COVID-19 among black and ethnic minority communities in England underlined the growing evidence that indicates people from black, Asian, and minority ethnic groups were at increased risk of mortality due to COVID-19 with a higher risk of transmission of infection due to the socio-economic conditions and the mortality due to underlying factors of co-morbidities.

Public Health England highlights the increased risk of exposure and acquisition due to barriers in accessing timely care and increased threats as a result of deprivation and discrimination people of Black, Asian and Ethnic minority groups face. Though the health inequalities are not new in the UK, the disparate effect of this infection brings back focus on the longstanding issues of the unjust and unnecessary gap in health outcomes experienced by the minority ethnic communities. Within the discourse of healthism, there is covert a tendency to blame victims for the health inequalities they suffer from. Media, in particular, pick up things out of context and reinforce stereotypes, demonizing cultural practices and behaviour of minority ethnic communities. Conversations are framed, reinforcing prejudicial views on health inequalities. From generalization that these communities do not 'take COVID seriously' to blaming people of Pakistani and Bangladeshi origin for living in 'crowded multigenerational households' without looking at the structural reason behind these compulsions. The poor health outcomes of Black, Asian and minority ethnic groups, have been there before the Covid −19 pandemic and manifested in a range of diseases and ailments. These inequalities range from a high risk of death during pregnancy to a higher risk of mental health issues, and a high prevalence of Type-2 Diabetes, hypertension, asthma, and coronary heart diseases. Drawing on the interrelation between the colonial past and a highly unequal present, Melania Calestani writes that disproportionate daily death tolls due to Covid-19 among Black, Asian and ethnic minority populations in the UK reveal the 'fault lines of social and economic exclusions' these people suffer from.

Health Inequalities

There is no single definition of health inequalities to understand the concept within varying socio-political contexts. A range of explanations have been put forward to conceptualise health inequalities with a focus on variations in the health achievements of individuals and groups' outcomes (Kawachi et al., 2002), differences in health status, disparities in health between rich and poor people (Graham, 2004), and unfair and unjust disparities within and between countries (Krieger, full reference), multidimensional social and economic disadvantage of ethnic minority people (Chouhan & Nazroo, 2020), The World Health Organisation puts health inequalities within the context of socially produced inequities in health which underline the systematic differences in health status between different social and economic groups. Here the focus is on inequities that create differences in health outcomes at a larger population level rather than at an individual level.

There are some definitions which go beyond explaining the phenomenon of health inequality to suggest ways of fighting it. Braveman (2016), focusing on equity and justice, argues for fairness and equal opportunity to address poverty, discrimination and empower people through better access to education, jobs, housing and health care. McCartney et al. (2019) analyzing a range of definitions and conceptualizations provide a more holistic view of health inequalities as the systematic, avoidable and unfair differences in health outcomes' seen between people, groups within the same population or as a 'gradient across a population ranked by social positions'.

In the United Kingdom, whether measured in terms of mortality, life expectancy or health status, health inequalities are increasing (Wilkinson, 1996, Nazroo, 2003; Yates-Doerr, 2020). Bambra et al. (2021) identify increased vulnerability, increased susceptibility, increased exposure and increased transmission as the four potential links between inequality and higher rates of Cvoid-19 infections. This conceptualization explains how socially deprived and economically disadvantaged communities of minority ethnic groups saw an increase in Covid cases.

There is a general understanding among the academics, policymakers and practitioners that inequalities in health are a direct result of the unequal society we live in. Socioeconomic factors like housing, education, employment, access to services gender, and ethnic background all play a part in determining health and wellbeing. The inequalities categorised by socio-economic measures and ethnic group or gender have also been linked with the areas people live in, and their racial, minority and immigration status (Adams, 1995a, b; Kawachi et al., 1997). Within the official discourse, the government documents also acknowledge this link between ethnicity, poverty and poor health. Along with low achievement in education, higher unemployment, poor housing and a higher rate of crime, poor health is also disproportionately prevalent among minority ethnic groups. When seen in combination with racism and discrimination, the racial background of people is seen as contributing to the illness (McKenzie, 2003).

Decades of epidemiological work have illustrated the socio-economic determinants of health and illness (Marmot & Wilkinson, 1999; Marmot & Siegrist, 2004). But most of the epidemiological work focuses on the social and material conditions including income overlooking the cultural and political aspects of life. It fails to appreciate the knowledge and experience of the people living on the margins. That perhaps is the reason, despite much of the epidemiological evidence, there is a lack of truly local data on health inequalities relating to ethnicities. Even the work of Richard G Wilkinson (1996), considered seminal in explaining health inequalities in the developed world, fails to engage with issues such as identity, faith and tradition in linking ethnicity with health and well-being. Writing about the social links between health and inequality he draws attention to the fact that social, rather than material, factors are the limiting component in the quality of life in developed societies. Using examples from the USA, Japan, Britain and Eastern Europe, he argues that there is a critical relationship between equality and health. He adds, 'the message that comes through clearly in each case is that the healthy, egalitarian countries have or had a sense of social cohesion and public spiritedness' (Wilkinson, 1996: 8). He argues that egalitarian societies with little disparities in income show lesser inequalities in health, while economically unequal societies are less stable socially with poor interaction, which reduced health and wellbeing. But there seems an inherent difficulty in mapping the ethnic epidemiological categories onto policy recommendations based on complex 'psycho-social and community-level phenomena and processes such as social identity and participation (Campbell & McLean, 2003). Inequality thus is not a fixed one-dimensional phenomenon, but a dynamic process involving power relations exercised through social, economic, cultural, and psychological processes. Many critical perspectives agree on the interplay of power and culture within the discourse of 'healthism' which has been described as an ideological construct wherein the responsibility of health is shifted from the individual to the state linking the public objectives of good health with the desire of an individual to stay well (Rose, 1999).

Health Inequalities Among Minority Communities

Ethnicity is a complex social construct that takes into account language, country of origin and shared traditions of people, where definitions often emerge from a subjective perspective of how people like to be identified as a group. Whatever way the term ethnicity is conceptualized, it becomes an indispensable part of policy discourse, especially when looking at the disparities and disadvantages ethnic minority groups face, mostly due to structural reasons. This disadvantage is reflected in many aspects of life, and the poor health outcomes of people belonging to Black and Asian Minority Ethnic groups demonstrate the health inequalities that exist and are increasing in the UK.

Though data is patchy, people from BAME report poor health and report a poor experience of using health services. People from minority ethnic groups especially Bangladeshi and Pakistani people have the poorest health outcomes. Similarly, infant and maternal mortality, diabetes and heart diseases are higher among these communities. People of South Asian origin show increased mortality from cardiovascular diseases and strokes. The mortality rate due to diabetes is also higher among people of South Asian origin. The risk of developing Type 2 diabetes among South Asian people is six times higher than in while groups with about 400,000 from South Asian groups accounting for one-fifth of the UK diabetes population.

There is a fund of literature available about the health disparities, especially among ethnic minority groups based on socio-economic conditions, geographic location and due to experiences of exclusion and racism (A, 1993; Coker, 2002). Covid 19 pandemic exhibited a more nuanced nature of these inequalities and has brought the issues to the centre stage once again. In one of the more startling studies, Nuffield Foundation-funded research undertaken by academics from the Universities of Sussex and Manchester has shown that as the people of Pakistani and Bangladeshi origin age, the health inequalities get wider to the white British population. The study reveals that after reaching 30, Pakistani and Bangladeshi people exhibit the worst health of any ethnic group, and the level of poor health among these groups matches that of White people 20 years older than them. This inequality gets worse when it comes to the health of women of Pakistani and Bangladeshi origin (Stopforth et al., 2021)

As mentioned before the Covid-19 pandemic revealed the extent of health inequalities, especially when it comes to minority ethnic communities. Though we are not fully out of the impact of this pandemic many studies have examined how Covid-19 amplified the gaps in health between people, geographies and cultures across the UK. Early studies bring to the surface the relationship between poor health and poverty, especially among the disadvantaged communities living in deprived areas (Bambra et al., 2021). As per the Ministry of Housing, Communities and Local Government's English Indices of Deprivation (2019), people from the Pakistani ethnic group are 3 times as likely as White British people to live in the most overall deprived areas in England. The index of multiple deprivation (IMD 2019) which takes into account 7 major types of dispositions based on the deprivation in income, Employment, Education, Health, Crime, Housing and Living environment), highlights that 31.1% of people of Pakistani origin 19.3% of Bangladeshi origin people are most likely to live in the most deprived areas. In contrast only 15.7% of other Asian people and just 9.0% of White people are likely to live in the most deprived areas in England. But this data needs to be put in the right context as people of Pakistani and Bangladeshi are disproportionately represented in these areas. The Covid-19 pandemic resulted in more deaths among Bangladeshi and Pakistani males and females. Besides the deprivation and disadvantage such groups face, other important issues are the structural racism and marginalization that contributes to health inequalities. Racism, which is now seen as growing as Islamophobia which results in discrimination is seen to harm the physical and mental health of the victims. A racist attitude also creates hurdles in accessing services. When seen in conjunction with a higher unemployment rate and poor housing, the inequality in health gets more entrenched to become a structural issue that needs to have a holistic approach than a clinical approach. Source: ONS (2021)

Discriminations and racism have been recognized as contributing factors to the exclusion of minorities which eventually leads to multiple deprivations and disadvantages for such groups (Weller et al., 2001). Discrimination based on affiliations to a religious group has grown in many public services in the UK (Sheridan, 2006). Islamophobia, a growing prejudice that leads to the discrimination of Muslim communities has been identified to lead to health inequalities. Despite obvious differences in the organisation, administration, funding and availability of health care in the UK National Health Service (NHS) and the US healthcare system, we argue that comparable societal forces of marginalisation and "faith-blind" or "religion-blind" health policies challenge the health of Muslim families and their access to culturally appropriate care. The use of Muslim identity and Islamic faith has remained ambiguous; being applied interchangeably between ethnic and racial groups.

Though identified as a limiting factor in tackling health inequalities, religious discrimination is seen hardly as an issue in policy and regulations due to the secular nature of the institutions and the fact religion is seen as a private affair of individuals (Laird et al., 2007). As such religious identity has remained out of any analysis to understand health inequalities. Though Sikhs and Jews were protected as ethnic minorities while Muslims as religious minorities remained unprotected under the Race Relations Act of 2000. The link between health and deprivation is substantiated by the fact that more deprived communities, living in clusters in poor neighbourhoods in the UK experience worse health with a shorter life expectancy than the groups who are better off and live in more developed areas. It is no surprise as 22 per cent of ethnic groups live in the most deprived areas. These facts, however, don't translate into public health policies as socioeconomic aspects of ethnicity and health outcomes remain on the margins of policy work (Chouhan & Nazroo, 2020).

The Covid-19 pandemic also affected this community disproportionately with these groups were found more likely to be diagnosed with Covid-19, get severely ill and die compared to the white population. Although not fully understood, there is a consensus among researchers, practitioners and policy makers that people belonging to Ethnic minority groups disproportionately face socio-economic deprivation, which is a key determinant of health and wellbeing in all communities. Similarly, structural racism is seen to reinforce inequalities having a negative impact on the physical and mental health of people from ethnic minority groups.

Arguing for a holistic approach to understanding the dynamics of health inequalities, Nazroo and Karlsen argue that ethnicity and health is mediated through structural factors, implying that the socio-economic situation, racism and discrimination should be part of any analysis that tries to explore the relationship between ethnicity and health inequality. (Nazroo & Karlsen, 2001:3). Suman Fernando (1991) dealing with issues of race in health says that race, culture and ethnicity can help in group identities like the post-slavery shaping of black consciousness in the US and the cultural revival of West Indian consciousness extending to other non-white groups living in the inner city ghettoes of the UK as a result of 'internal colonialism', 'collective class action' which is seen a source 'social stability', place of 'mutual support, and homeliness' (Hall et al., 1978; Pryce, 1979; Castells, 1983; Revill, 1993; Bauman, 2000). Being together is thus necessitated by the fact that a complex discourse of being non-white and being represented differently (Hall, 1997), originating from former British colonies (Barrera, 1979:194), creates a discourse of racialisation and 'othering' people. This discourse creates a culture of exclusion which is further aggravated by the barriers to access and participation (Hardill et al., 2001). These experiences take people towards community, which provides both a refuge and a means to contest exclusion (Jeffery, 1976:182). But as discussed at some length in Chap. 4 of this thesis, the community is a highly complex construct, and this study sees it more as a position and strategy to negotiate commonalities and differences.

In a multiracial and multicultural society concept of ethnicity, identified by a sense of belonging emerges through various pressures, social, political, economic etc. as well as cultural toes and perception of racial identity, the strength of which too may be influenced by these pressures. Among the social forces in many societies is the pressure arising from racism that drives together people perceived as being racially similar to each other…This is the ethnicity that is of practical importance in most communities where there is racial and cultural diversity. However, if, in any such society, the significance of racism diminishes, cultural difference is likely to achieve increasing importance in determining ethnicity. But while racism continues, as it does in most Western societies, racial difference plays an important part in determining ethnicity (1991: 15I).

Healthism and Governmentality

The growing managerialism in the National Health Services is perceived by many as evidence of the shift from Socialism to laissez-faire thinking where the role of the market is seen as central to the health policy, changing it from service to power (Greener, 1999). The role of the NHS is in conflict with the public beliefs of what service is about and how it should work. Learmonth (1997), surveying the public attitudes towards managerialism in the NHS, writes managers 'attempt to control' organisations to make them 'efficient', is seen as a neo-Taylorist response to 'perceived failures in the service' and justified as part of 'New Right ideology'. The obsession 'with value for money' and setting targets to achieve it is perceived by the general public as conflicting with a 'service for individual care' (Ibid.: 215). This growth in managerialism, characterised by efficiency, target setting, rewards and penalties has created an environment in which every health professional is feeling under pressure to perform to the standards set by managers. Within this environment, every member of staff becomes a tool to deliver. He/She loses the human touch. The cultural, social and other backgrounds of staff become immaterial as one is sucked into this new culture of managerialism.

The National Health Service (NHS) operates in a very difficult situation, and one cannot overlook the issues of under-funding and higher public expectations, but adding layers of bureaucracies does not help either. Many argue that the NHS needs to acknowledge a holistic approach to dealing with inequalities. In this regard, the lack of awareness and knowledge of the culture and how to deal with respect and dignity impact the health of those the NHS wants to help. Racial prejudice and discrimination affect people directly and the health services in many areas are inappropriate and insensitive to the culture and beliefs of patients (Balarajan & Raleigh, 1995; Smaje, 1995; Acheson, 1998; Modood, 1997; Nazroo, 1997). The NHS's focus on tailoring services to perceived needs does not take into account a patient's health beliefs and knowledge. Free and McKee (1998) highlight this cultural inadequacy in service provision when it comes to serving non-white minority groups.

In the Health Survey for England conducted by the National Centre for Social Research and the Department of Epidemiology and Public Health at the Royal Free and University College Medical School in 1999, it was found that among the adult male population of minority ethnic groups, Pakistani, Bangladeshi and Irish, limiting longstanding illness was 30 to 65 per cent higher than for men in the general population (Erens et al., 1999). Pakistani and Bangladeshi men and women were seen as three to four times more likely than the general population to rate their health as bad or very bad. The psychosocial health of Bangladeshi and Pakistani men and women was seen as scoring high on the General Health Questionnaire (GHQ12) (A high score on this is an indicator of possible psychiatric morbidity). The general practitioner (GP) consultations were observed to be higher for South Asian and Afro-Caribbean men (Erens et al., 1999).

It is interesting to look at the pattern of the response from the health services to address this issue. Overall, the response has been to offer interpreters, and translators and provide for the religious and cultural needs of the non-white population, e.g. the display of leaflets in Hindi/Urdu, and Punjabi at surgeries. This attitude of creating specialised services does not help in mainstreaming services. This approach to improving the health of minority ethnic groups is in a way asking service users to change and adapt to the way of service providers (Mocroft et al., 1999). However, the NHS is not a homogenous organisation. There are people from different racial backgrounds, nationalities and ethnicities working for this organization, making it one of the most racially diverse services in the UK, employing more than 1.3

million staff, the largest employer in Europe serving over 50 million people in England alone. The NHS claims to have equality and diversity at the heart of its strategy by investing in the NHS workforce to deliver a better service and improve patient care. This is very critical for an organisation, which serves over 50 million people in England. This richness within the NHS is seen as an asset and potential for addressing the health needs of the diverse people it serves.

The covid-19 pandemic did shake the very core of health services but at the same time, it woke up politicians and policymakers to the need of running NHS within the ethos of social justice to address the ugly health inequalities the pandemic exposed. We are witnessing a cross-party push to break from the 'governing sensibilities' of the last 30 years. These sensibilities dominated by increasing competition were fundamentally against the founding principle of equality and social justice. From public to private to PPP, the NHS's journey is marred with policies and decisions political in nature and ideological in content. Both the Conservative and the Labour governments have played political football to score points while the core responsibility of serving people became a victim of managerialism, governmentality and racialization. As public service reform remains elusive, the Covid-19 pandemic has revealed the ugly truth of unacceptable health inequalities that still exist in the UK. In this context, Dutta, Lovering and Knafo in their Editorial comment in Tribune (March 2021) argue for restoring power to doctors and nurses from managers and bureaucrats.

Going back to how NHS reached the current situation, we need to look back at the studies, and inquiries commissioned by successive governments since the 70's to reform National Health Service. Several reports and White Papers have been published but here we will briefly discuss some important ones which have impacted the Health Services most.

Black Report

Health Inequality in the UK is not a new issue. Way back in 1977, the Labour government commissioned a Working Group chaired by Sir Douglas Black to find differences in mortality rates, and access to health services, especially among those coming from lower social groups and working classes. The report which was published in 1980 suggested addressing broader social issues like improving living and working conditions, providing higher child benefit, and strengthening community and primary care through increased government interventions. With power shifting to Conservatives did not implement these recommendations. NHS (and other) public service reforms have been dominated by a market approach since the late 1980s under successive Conservative, Labour and Coalition (Conservative and Liberal Democrat) Governments. Few strong doubts about them made their way into official documents until the late 2010s. Indeed, some, but not all, dimensions of markets, particularly perhaps the shift from administrative service agreements to legally binding contracts, have become embedded in the NHS and are now taken for granted.

Our task has been to review the evidence on inequalities in health in England, including time trends, and, as a contribution to the development of the Government's strategy for health, to identify areas for policy development likely to reduce these inequalities. We carried out our task over the last 12 months, drawing on scientific and expert evidence, and peer review. Although average mortality has fallen over the past 50 years, unacceptable inequalities in health persist. For many measures of health, inequalities have either remained the same or have widened in recent decades. These inequalities affect the whole of society and they can be identified at all stages of the life course from pregnancy to old age. The weight of scientific evidence supports a socioeconomic explanation of health inequalities. This traces the roots of ill health to such determinants as income, education and employment as well as to the material environment and lifestyle. It follows that our recommendations have implications across a broad front and reach far beyond the remit of the Department of Health. Some relate to the whole Government while others relate to particular Departments. We have identified a range of areas for future policy development, judged on the scale of their potential impact on health inequalities, and the weight of evidence.

These areas include poverty, income, tax and benefits; education; employment; housing and environment; mobility, transport and pollution; and nutrition. Areas are also identified by the stages of the life course – mothers, children and families; young people and adults of working age; and older people – and by focusing on ethnic and gender inequalities. We identify possible steps within the National Health Service to reduce inequalities. In our view, these areas offer opportunities over time to improve the health of the less well off. There are three areas which we regard as crucial: all policies likely to have an impact on health should be evaluated in terms of their impact on health inequalities; a high priority should be given to the health of families with children; further steps should be taken to reduce income inequalities and improve the living standards of poor households.

Acheson Report

When Labour came to power after a landslide win in 1997, the then health secretary Tessa Jowel constituted an independent inquiry into health inequalities under Sir Donald Acheson to identify trends in health inequalities, and set priority areas for policy development for government intervention and to develop a new strategy for health. The report published in 1998, analysed the data from the Office of National Statistics, Department of Health and other sources, and highlighted the socioeconomic dimension of health inequalities tracing reasons for ill-health to income, education and employment along with lifestyle and conditions under which they live. The inquiry recommended 'poverty, income, tax and benefits; education; employment; housing and environment; mobility, transport and pollution; and nutrition' as key areas for policy development to address health inequalities. The commission suggested priority be given to the health of families with children, reduce inequalities in income and improve the living conditions of the people.

NHS Reform from 1980

The last three decades have seen NHS being driven more and more towards market-based reforms, which has created this consumer/providers binary with competition being prioritized for these tax-funded services. The Health and Social Care Act of 2012 provided the legislative power to this service with a significant impact that gave more hand to politicians, managers and medical professionals. Lewis writes that the three decades of market approach to the delivery of health services in the UK exhibited a 'continuity between Conservatives and Labour in respect of means, mechanisms and often short term policy goals'. Lewis adds that while Labour talked about 'choice', Conservatives based their arguments in favour of the market and less interference by the state. Traditionally Labour has promised to address health inequalities, and after the recommendation of the Acheson report, it focused on the implementation of health inequalities measures from 1998 to 2010. This strategy was designed to support families, increase access to healthcare; and tackle social determinants of health. As a result of these strategies and actions, there was an improvement in reducing health inequalities but New Labours' obsession with league tables led to the creation of new bureaucracies and red tape. The impact is understood to have been better had the policy focus not moved more towards 'life-style drift, highlighting the individual-level behaviour rather than working on social determinants. There was less emphasis on tackling economic inequality and more on changing people's behaviour. Consequently, healthism and governmentality have become a norm, and the concepts gained more currency during the New Labour rule which was obsessed with a managerial approach to public services. This managerial approach to health services is seen as taking a more mechanistic view of inequalities in health, ignoring the structural and cultural perspectives

In the first chapter of this book, we explored how the discourse of social exclusion is managed by bureaucracies and regimes that problematise 'otherness' and abnormalize spaces (Levitas, 1998; Shah, 1998). This 'managed' conceptualisation of disadvantage and deprivation has led to the emergence of a 'managerial state'-businesslike organising, providing and delivery of welfare by increasing efficiency through the setting of targets and hiring more managers (Clarke, 1992). The government strategies to 'manage' the dynamics of internal diversity are seen by many scholars as part of the New Labour's shift from welfare to a more neo-liberal agenda. The obsession with marketisation, audits and targets has been criticised for being too managerial, centralised and serving the interests of capital (Penna, 2004). These scholars find the Labour government's public service reform characterised by the rhetoric of choice, voice, responsibility and empowerment, a continuation of the Thatcherite project of abandonment of the citizen through the dismantling of the protections constructed in post-war welfare capitalism against the vagaries, demands and inequities of the market and the unconstrained powers of capital (2004: 450).

In the name of efficiency, effectiveness and performance, many areas of public life, especially services are becoming increasingly the subject of managerial hegemony. Phrases such as 'medical' and 'governance' have become an integral part of the health policy, illustrating New Labour's obsession with a narrow clinical understanding of health and well-being, on the one hand, and an increased reliance on the processes of 'managing' health on the other. The official definition of clinical governance is given in the NHS circular, Clinical Governance: Quality in the New NHS17. Michael Purdy (1999) argues that the central feature of the strategy to endorse the medical view of health is to make individuals, families and communities responsible for their health/ ill health. He says that this process of shifting responsibility makes people 'police themselves and declare their membership of the nation, through their healthy lifestyles', making health a 'component of citizenship'. Looking at the Conservative government's strategy (The Health of the Nation DOH 1992) and the Labour government's (Our Healthier Nation, DOH 1998), Purdy contextualises these policies within the neo-liberal and neo-conservative perspectives and finds many similarities between the two.

The Labour government policy documents acknowledge the social, economic and environmental causes of ill health, which it thinks require a partnership between governments, communities and individuals to deal with. However, Purdy (1999), remarks that despite the government's desire to 'narrow the health gap', New Labour's strategy has not made the fight against health inequalities part of the national priority. He argues the by emphasis the socially 'responsible choice', New Labour echoes and endorses the neo-conservative theme of the individual's responsibility to society. He believes that 'healthism', which can exclude those who need public health measures most, focuses more on health policies related to 'lifestyle management'. This process he sees marginalizing those who, due to a variety of social, economic and cultural reasons, suffer from poor health. The discourse of healthism, linking health with citizenship and emphasizing lifestyle management and the responsible behaviour of people, is believed to create subjectivities (Lupton, 1995), which are governed through 'new forms of social regulation' (Bunton, 1992). Health promotion thus becomes a tool of such regulation as it is used to raise awareness about 'guarding the self' as a responsible citizen:

> *In effect, the health promotion strategies such as the Health of the Nation (1992) and our Healthier Nation (1998) construct health in such a way as to exclude sections of the population... The risk there is that different and minority lifestyles that do not fit cleanly into the healthy norm may become seen as deviant, undesirable and even dangerous. Moreover, the privileging of health as a cultural norm and equating it with rational behaviour denies the cultural validity of alternative discourses to that of health promotion.* (Bunton, 1992: 72–73)

Sue Penna (2004) takes this debate further by suggesting that it is 'unhelpful to see policy formulation in purely national terms' against the backdrop of the UK's increased involvement in regional, international and global networks of governance and regulatory framework, which create a 'new legal regime' with a 'neo-liberal policy agenda'. Citing the examples of the UK membership of the European Union

(EU), International Monetary Fund (IMF) and World Trade Organisation (WTO), Penna argues that these regimes define the 'the parameters for domestic policy in important ways' and produce much of the social exclusion it purports to address by keeping social welfare out of the policy discourses (2004:2). Calling the process of managing people's lives a discourse of 'governmentality', Clarke, J. (2005: 453) from a Foucauldian analysis, argues that this process 'seeks to transform citizens into subjects' who understand themselves as responsible and independent agents. He adds that activation, empowerment, responsibilization and abandonment constitute four dynamics of the process of governmentality, of which 'New Labour appears as exemplary practitioners'. Clarke finds the 'revelatory style' of Foucauldian analysis helpful in uncovering the complex and subtle workings of power. The production of self-regulating subjects such as job seekers, marginalised, inner-city dwellers, illegal immigrants, hard-working families, socially excluded and so on are categories used to manage diversity (2005: 454).

Such an approach not only serves as a convenient means of categorisation that essentialise difference, but is also used as a pretext to pass the blame of exclusion on to the victims of inequality. A variety of rhetoric has become a part of New Labour's strategy to be seen as 'doing something', which includes listening, enabling, activating and making people responsible for their actions and their duties. Clarke (2005) analyses this approach and finds that participatory governance is 'structurally, rarely integrated with other governance institutions or processes and often disconnected from consequences or outcomes'. This analysis further finds out that activation is a process of making people into 'market-ready' workers, empowerment a mask to conceal the 'systematic stripping of forms of power and protection' of welfare embodied in social citizenship, and responsibility a smokescreen to hide the responsibilities of the state. Clarke argues that the only real thing in New Labour's rhetoric of change and reform is the abandonment of citizens to the 'advantage of capital in its global and local forms' (Ibid: 453).

The abandonment of social justice by New Labour in favour of markets makes many commentators believe that the NHS has a dangerous future under it. Purdy and Banks (1999) believe that New labour's 'third way' – promising continuity with neo-conservatism but distancing itself from neo-liberal individualism, will abandon principles of equity and universal coverage by the health service and thereby extend the experience of exclusion. The third-way emphasis on local consultation and partnerships to decentralise control could also mean that the central government is abdicating its responsibility (Purdy & Banks, 1999: 16–19). While many government discourses talk about empowerment to fight exclusion and give people the opportunity to take control, in reality, the process of empowerment is not that simple. Empowerment is more than social change, it is a process of undoing internalized oppression (Nagar & Raju, 2003).

The notion of empowerment is linked to the condition of disempowerment and refers to a process of change by which people acquire the ability to make choices. It demands both an agency and structural approach to emphasise both education and addressing power inequalities, the ownership of which can change the structural inequalities (Kabeer, 1999). The abuse of the structural, institutional and professional power, which has made people silent and dependent, cannot be simply changed by asking excluded people to fill in the form and tick boxes. The provider-lead models can work only so far as people are co-opted into managerial exercises.

Embedded in this process of governmentality, health is linked not only to well-being but to citizenship and nationhood. In the health policy discourse, such phrases and terms as 'responsible citizens', 'healthy people making good choices' and 'our healthier nation' reinforce this process of activation and responsibilisation. For Clarke et al. (2000:110) these citizens are, as a growing body of Foucauldian scholarship indicates, the subjects of practices of the governmental constitution. In particular, they are not just responsible; 'they are the product of processes of responsibilization'. Part of this managerial practice consists of borrowing concepts and ideas and adapting them in a way to put gloss and spin on the government's failure to deal with structural reasons that lead to inequalities. Paul Bagguley and Yasmin Hussain (2003) illustrate this phenomenon by examining the discourse of community cohesion and segregation used in three Home office-sponsored reports (Cantle, Denham and Ritchie) on the 2001 riots in the northern English towns of Bradford, Burnley and Oldham. They argue that these reports were written within a general context in which the discourses of the community were sought in support of government goals.

Need for a Holistic Approach

The 1986 Ottawa Charter of the World Health Organisation (WHO) defined health promotion as the 'process of enabling people to increase control over and to improve their health'. This approach in enabling and facilitating peoples' participation in health improvement with a focus on increased awareness, self-responsibility and adopting healthy lifestyles has become a mantra of all public health policies. The empowerment strategies of the National Health Services in the UK have long been advocated for addressing health inequalities especially for vulnerable and 'powerless' groups of people, mostly minority ethnic groups. In all health promotion strategies, the fundamental focus has been on providing the relevant information about services, rights and responsibilities through appropriate means concerning cultural sensitivities of people. What remains to be seen is if in reality people, especially those who live on the margins of society, are involved in decisions about their health and well-being and if can exercise informed choices. Liz Kendall (2001) argues for a more participatory health care system:

> *For too long, healthcare systems have treated patients as passive recipients and given them little information or say regarding how and by whom they are cared for. Although health system reformers have rightly sought to expand patient choice, they have not given the same weight to what patients should be expected to do in return. Good health is the responsibility not just of governments, doctors, and nurses, but also of people themselves. To improve health, we must go beyond merely treating disease, to transforming the relationship among doctors, patients, and their health services. We must move from a purely consumerist model*

of healthcare to a citizenship model in which patients have more rights and choices, but in which they also take on greater responsibility. (Kendall, 2001: 58–59)

Kendall echoes the Labour government's emphasis on the communitarian approach, which has come under severe criticism for shifting responsibilities to the victims of inequalities and exclusion. Many studies have, however, highlighted the fact that initiatives for empowering people in marginalized communities should understand and address the complexity of social and cultural experiences and attitudes in these communities (Zimmerman & Rapport, 1988). These communities, however, are not homogenous but show heterogeneity and variations based on caste, village loyalty and family kinship. It is debated that among the dynamics affecting the efficiency and outcomes of health promotion is the relevance and appropriateness of the person's community and cultural background. Many research projects (Fernando, 1991) especially within ethnic, indigenous and aboriginal groups the world over, suggest that the Western approaches to the health of marginalized people need refocusing and restructuring to accommodate appropriate approaches which complement faith, tradition and the way of life of these groups. Identity, ethnicity and spirituality are too important dimensions of the life of minority groups to be ignored in any health promotion and intervention.

In the UK, the wider marginalisation of non-white people by the public institutions and services is also true in the case of health services. Although the Human Rights Act 1998 and the Race Relations (Amendment) Act 2000 place responsibilities on service providers to eradicate discriminatory procedures and practices, the DoH acknowledges the inequitable variation in the use of health care services between ethnic groups. (Acheson, 1998; Department of Health and Sir Donald Acheson, 1998). Similarly, the Race Relations (Amendment) Act (2000) places a duty on public authorities to actively promote race equality and it requires that listed organizations have a race equality scheme. Health and social care agencies have a statutory duty to eliminate unlawful discrimination and to demonstrate evidence such as monitoring the effects of policies on ethnic minority groups, training and setting race equality objectives. In his editorial comment, Richard Smith (1999: 90), quoting Tudor Hart's famous paper on —the inverse care law, argues that medicine fails the marginalized. Hart's law suggests that those who need medical care the most are the least likely to get it. It is not just the stark disparities in health between the poor living in the developed and developing world, but that, as Smith argues, evidence continues to accumulate that the law applies everywhere, and things are probably getting worse not better. Looking at the health inequalities, it can be said that health services in the UK, no doubt are the best in the world, fail poor, vulnerable and those who are marginalized. Smith cites possible reasons for this failure such as a 'combination of ignorance, fear, and prejudice plus a feeling that they should adapt to the services rather than the other way around' (1999:1589–1590).

Based on these reports, recommendations and general policy interventions, several initiatives have been taken to improve the health of people living in deprived city areas and address the wider issue of inequality in health. After decades of inaction, the introduction of multi-agency initiatives, including 'Sure Start', Health

Action Zone (HAZ), Healthy Living Centres (HLCs) and Health Improvement Programme (HimP) in the late '90 s was seen to step in the right direction to develop a bottom-up approach. The New Public Health agenda highlighted the need for improvement in health through organised interventions directed at the public or the community level (DoH, 1998). Addressing health issues through the action zone has emerged as one of the key characteristics of New Labour's approach. This may be part of the New Labour's third-way approach, but many of the unresolved problems have resurfaced, as has the debate on whether health inequality can be dealt with at the place level or the people level? (Moon & Powell, 2001: 43).

But these initiatives led to a greater willingness to involve the community/voluntary sector in activities mainly to do with the health of black and minority ethnic groups. Mocroft et al. (1999) observe several activities wherein this sector is used for service delivery, translation, interpretation, information provision, education, and advocacy services, besides the outreach support, local research into needs, community development and informal counselling services. But the use of community and voluntary groups in health promotion can be problematic due to a lack of capacity to deal with complex issues, non-representative character, and lack of funding and resources (Sue, 1999). But the biggest problem in such initiatives is sustainability, as the government still adopts an ad hoc approach (Mocoroft et al., 1999). Involvement in and ownership of health initiatives have long been advocated for empowering communities to express and address their health needs. Wallerstein (1992) sees empowerment as a strategy for 'improving a population's health' and powerlessness as a 'risk factor for disease.' Most of the communitarian arguments, drawing support from the World Health Organization (WHO) policy, take a holistic rather than a 'narrow clinical approach' to health promotion which is seen as a shift from educationist bio-medical models of avoiding ill-health and taking personal responsibility to a more emancipatory view of health and its determinants (Whitehead, 1987). Although health promotion through participatory action research has been used for some time in the developing world, especially in India and among the aboriginals, indigenous and minority groups in Australia, New Zealand and Canada (Bhandari & Mills, 2003; Fleming & Parker, 2001), there is very little evidence of such an approach being used within Europe and the UK.

In a world of renewed interest in civil society and individual empowerment, health is seen as more than a disease-free condition. Self-determination and human rights have entered into the domain of health and the influence of cultural, social and philosophical aspects including the spiritual dimensions – meaning and purpose of life and the quality of relationships are seen as the key determinant in health and wellbeing (Ryff & Singer, 1998). But many scientists find such a connection absurd. The research into the role of spirituality in health is argued to be methodologically weak, with a deficiency in data and often biased. Much of the literature on faith and health is based on the somatic principle that religious affiliation and membership benefit health by promoting healthy behaviour and lifestyles. If this principle is convincing enough to help people stay healthy, then does this mean people should get membership in a religious group to be healthier? But people do not become religious to stay healthy; People have different reasons, motivations and convictions to practice religion (Levin, 2001).

Empowerment Narrative

Literature from multiple domains and disciplines suggests that community empowerment, as a process of developing the capabilities of socially excluded and disadvantaged groups, should provide control over the actions and decisions that are detrimental to their health and wellbeing. Though the concepts of an empower-centred approach to equality, fairness and universal access to health and wellbeing is enshrined in numerous policies and declaration (WHO, 1986, 1998), there is a widening gulf between the policies and actual practices in many parts of the world. Scholars have time and again underlined the need for the collective control of communities as an important determinant of health equity (Wallerstein & Duran, 2006; Whitehead et al., 2016). For social and community development, community empowerment has now become an important part of community empowerment as is reflected in many local, national and international strategies for social and health development, including Global Sustainable Development Goal (Powell et al., 2021) Behavioural orientation is seen to be dependent on cultural resources which through a process of socialization leads to lifestyles and choices people make. Scholars argue for a more culture-centric approach in addressing inequalities in health and well being, especially the problems related to lifestyle.

Within the universe of this research, predominately South Asian, which is predominantly Muslim, the issue of faith and spirituality is an important dimension of their identity. Among these people, it has been observed that family kinships, community life and spiritual experience play an important part in the day to day existence. So, well-being entails the interplay of social and cultural relationships, and acknowledgement of these factors is indispensable for any health promotion. An understanding and appreciation of the subjective experience of minority ethnic people, particularly their relationship with spirituality, will help in more effective and empowering ways of encouraging people to take control and make more informed choices about their health and well-being. There has not been any systematic research done into the role faith and cultural practices can play in health education, but anecdotal evidence suggests that many mosques and community centres in the UK are becoming more proactive in addressing issues of health inequality. The NHS has been working with religious groups in inner-city areas to help people give up smoking. But there are issues around sustainability as the NHS is not institutionally getting involved with faith groups on a long term basis in addressing the issues of health inequality. However, the private sector in certain instances has already made some inroads into the Muslim community through mosques. The Roche HealthCare Company worked with London's Islamic Cultural Centre to raise awareness about a variety of health concerns, such as type 2 Diabetes, Coronary heart disease and other obesity-related illnesses, specifically targeting London's Muslim community. About 700 people attended the three-day event (Muslim Council of Britain). Dr. Shuja Shafi, Consultant Microbiologist, Health Protection Agency Collaborating Laboratory, North West London Hospitals NHS Trust and Chairman of Health & Medical Committee of the Muslim Council of Britain commented:

> *The Government is addressing Diabetes and Coronary heart disease through National Service Frameworks which aim to improve health and reduce inequalities, but there is a lot the Muslim community can do for themselves to increase awareness, educate and empower people to make informed decisions about their lifestyle and health. A focused event such as this one, held in collaboration between the Mosque and a healthcare company provides an excellent example of what can be achieved to reach the diverse Muslim community comprising different ethnic groups.* (MCB, 2003)

The role of spirituality especially the Islamic concept of Health and well-being is not well understood within the Eurocentric literature. Many epidemiological studies to see if there is a religious factor in health have shown that there is very little appreciation of religion and spirituality in health and disease management (Levin & Schiller, 1987). The view from the community is that the government is ignoring the experiences and knowledge of those it tries to improve. With a general disregard for non-Western points of view, the attitude of health professionals and their managers is seen as not sensitive and appropriate, as is clearly explained by one of the interviewees Haji Ishaq (HI):

> *Prayers have a powerful effect on one's health. Our daily life and routine are dictated by praying...it gives me strength in old age. But do these healthy people accept this...No I do not think so! They try to find medical reasons and remedies for everything, but we see illness and recovery as part of our fate and test of our endurance.*

Emphasizing the cross-cultural conception of illness, Fernando (1991) argues that Western tradition has excluded many non-Western ways of understanding illness. Arguing for distinction of disease from illness, and taking out the externalising/internalising binary, Fernando finds Western biomedical concepts of illness inadequate because of non-Western worldviews, which see disease and illness beyond biological aetiology. Alternative conceptions of illness are important in settings where cultural differences take the shape of racism. In the UK, the pre-conceived notions, prejudices and stereotyping of non-white people taint the way their illness is understood and treated. The lifestyle and cultural practices of these people are often seen as an aberration to the 'norm', and in many cases, the disease is racialised. In the process, anything non-Western is inferior and the scientific system is better than the traditional ways. Fernando finds this attitude of excluding non-Western culture type of a 'cultural blindness' resulting from racist behaviour. He further says that Western conceptions of illness are rooted in scientific reasoning which sees a person in isolation from his social, cultural and environmental factors, thereby rejecting the non-scientific dimensions of faith and knowledge that are integral to human experience.

The Cartesian-Newtonian framework on which the Western biomedical conception of health and illness is grounded has a strong secular bias because of its scientific and body-mind dualism. Writing against the backdrop of criticism of the Western mechanistic view of life, Fernando (1991), relying on Capra's (1982) systems approach to health and health care, argues for a holistic way consistent with cultural heritage and not necessarily averse to the spiritual traditions. This approach advocated by Freire (1972) stresses pedagogy through which one creates his reality from the circumstances of daily existence. Using the concept of banking education, he says that the more passive people are, the more they will adapt, the more their creativity will diminish and their naivety increase, which creates the conditions necessary for the oppressors to emerge as generous benefactors. This paradigm of empowerment lends support to the study in exploring how marginalized groups can use culture and tradition as a resource for empowerment. This process of realizing local and communal strengths and using them to promote people-centred initiatives can make peoples' participation real and meaningful (Fals-Borda, 1979; Freire, 1972). Religion, culture and community life become a significant part of this process and various conflicting perspectives come together in a creative way to address issues of marginalisation.

Where Do We Go from Here?

We need to have a better understanding of the determinants that lead to health inequalities among minority ethnic groups. Reliable data on social, cultural, structural, and economic factors can help to improve the health outcomes of these groups. The best way to achieve this goal is to involve the communities through participatory research to rebuild trust and empower people. Based on this data develop campaigns, especially in association with faith-based groups, to enhance efforts with culturally competent health promotion and disease prevention programmes especially targeting the common health issues like Diabetes, hypertension, Asthma, Coronary heart diseases, obesity, smoking cessation, and mental health. Need to understand data within the context of the living conditions and experiences of minority ethnic groups. This means facilitating, engaging and empowering people in developing ways and means to address health inequalities. The top-down model has not worked. The change has to come from within and a non-patronizing and fully resourced support from outside can develop better ways to address the issues.

Many people have lost their dear and near ones, and there is a trust deficit between people and the health services. While rebuilding this trust, the provision of high quality, culturally sensitive and socially appropriate and caring health care is developed. Cultural competence means providing holistic services that address social, faith, cultural, and linguistic needs. This competence is critical to address health of people of minority ethnic groups, who whom faith plays a big part in their lives. In practice, however, there is little or no engagement between service providers and faith groups which are very influential in local communities. While such groups played a critical role during Covid 19 pandemic by providing spiritual and community support to the victims, service providers operated in isolation to reinforce the clinical underpinnings of health services and stay away from the cultural and spiritual aspects of health and wellbeing.

There is an urgent need for a comprehensive framework that recognizes the role of community empowerment in improving the health outcomes of minority ethnic groups. The role of faith and cultural practices is of paramount importance in this framework as Muslims make one of the largest minority ethnic groups in the UK with a network of faith-based organisations including mosques, charities, schools, funeral services etc. The transformation of health care culture is an important goal, not only for Muslim patients but for patients of all religious backgrounds. However, as a key case study, health care research needs to focus attention on the specific experiences and health outcomes of Muslim youth, particularly in the current political and social context. Health narratives and the lived experiences of marginalised Muslims must inform culturally appropriate services.

Chapter 6
Contextual Approach to Communication

Local media can create a coherent narrative of a region's development and help people formulate goals and plans for how to improve their situation. The media can help contextualize national development programs within community frameworks and bring these goals closer to their intended beneficiaries. (UNESCO)

Community Media: A Common Frame of Reference

Bringing agency to the forefront, becomes important to validate voices from peripheries through participation, reflection and action. This does not mean that periphery can become centre, but opens up the possibility of recognizing other ways of living and being human. So, participation through the cultural practices and communal activities is seen critical to addressing social, cultural and economic conditions. Within the perspectives of alternative approaches in promoting marginalized points of view, a more contextual approach, where identity and representation facilitate participation, is seen more empowering for those living on peripheries of the mainstream. This study, researched and written within the paradigm of empowerment, explores the role a community based broadcasting initiative can play in providing a familiar, experiential and enabling context to this process. It benefits from the ethnographic study of a small-scale and community-based radio station – *Radio Ramzan* in inner city Nottingham to support the egalitarian link between people's experiences and expression.

The study remains very pertinent to the current debate on how Covid-19 has widened the stark inequalities in the health outcomes of the privileged groups and those are socially disadvantaged and live in the deprived inner city areas of Post-industrial towns in England. The radio station set up during *Ramadan* – the month of fasting in Islamic calendar, provided an environment for communal and spiritual awakening with talk shows, interviews, music and discussions to creating a dynamic

F. Malik, *Addressing Health Inequalities through Community Media*, https://doi.org/10.1007/978-3-031-35237-9_6

between experience, place, faith and media. Within this framework, the empowerment is linked to the democratic communication (this framework is explained in Chap. 4).

Within the gamut of alternative media, one of the most cost-effective means that has been used for decades in poor parts of the world, and is now getting popular among the marginalized communities in the West is the community radio. As Hartley (2000:153) puts it, 'radio continues to be used in a variety of community-building developmental situations, providing remote, marginal and disenfranchised communities with low-cost, low-tech public space'. Many scholars see community based radio playing a critical role in making communication a two-way process that can empower, increase participation and encourage local ownership of media (Barlow 1988, McQuail 1994; Couldry, 1999). Community radio is envisaged to provide a ground of 'communicative interaction' and serve as a 'frame of reference for shared interpretation' within a community (Hollander, 1992: 8). The first community stations began broadcasting over fifty years ago in Latin America. This sector of broadcasting has developed steadily since in various parts of the world. The community radio exists in a wide variety of forms throughout the world. The variety in names and definitions of these means of communication are 'not only due to linguistic differences but are also based on ideological and conceptual distinctions' (Prehn, 1992, 256). There are many common strands in these media. All such media are small scale in operation, mostly non-profit making with politically or ideologically committed editorial policy and action-oriented focus. These radios have a shared interest in representing and promoting marginalised points of view.

In the UK the government started experimenting with community broadcasting in 1985. The Green paper published in this regard stated: —community radio should be introduced throughout the UK, finding its place side by side with the existing local commercial station||. Despite the Minister of State's pledges to provide 200–300 additional local radio services, the Broadcasting Act of 1990 made no specific provision for community radio. The Act provided for Restricted Service Licenses (RSLs) for radio, allowing services for a particular establishment or other defined location, or a particular event, in the UK. However, the Radio Authority, the they either broadcast to a specific interest group – e.g. ethnic or language group; classical music; education – or provide programmes for sections of the community not properly catered for by Government and Commercial stations. From 1991 till the end of 1999, the Radio Authority now (Ofcom) had issued 2585 such licenses to various groups and people in different parts of the UK. The community broadcasting has since organized better in the UK with many groups and members of civil society lending support to the idea of creating a third tier of broadcasting in the country. One of the influential pressure groups that have been spearheading a campaign for community based radio in the UK is the 'Community Media Association', which has now developed into a one window shop for supporting and building capacity of community organizations interested in using radio for community development.[1] The surge in the demand for radio broadcasting licenses from community, religious and non-governmental organisations is a clear indication of the need and demand for a broadcasting structure outside the mainstream provisions. Among the

Restricted Service License (RSL) is a growing number of Radio Ramadan's which broadcast during the month of Ramadan in the Islamic calendar. The number of such station was six in 1994 which reached to 18 in 2000. While the main focus of these stations remains complementing religious duties during the month of fasting, an aim to provide an alternative vision of life and politics drives most of these stations.

Living as Ethnic Minority in a Poor Neighbourhood

Looking at the Ministry of Housing, communities and Local Government's deprivation data, based on Income, Employment, Health, Education, Crime, Housing and Living Environment, Nottingham ranks 10th most deprived local authorities in England. The Ministry and its predecessor has been compiling this data since 1970 to map the deprivation in some of the poorest neighbourhoods in England, and Nottingham has not shown much progress with 30 percent of children living in income-deprived families according to the Ministry's IoD2019 report. People from minority ethnic communities are disproportionately represented within these pockets of deprivations, with around fifty-six per cent living in the 44 most deprived local authorities in England. As per the 2011 Census, there are 35.6 per cent Black and Ethnic minority people living in Nottingham of which 13.1 per cent Asian, 16.9 per cent Black, 18.0 per cent mixed ethnic background and 29.8 percent other ethnic groups. Of the 35.6 per cent Asian population, most of the people are of South Asian- Mirpuri origin who are predominately Muslim. The majority of the Muslim community living in the Hyson Green, Lenton and Sneinton areas of Nottingham City the city have developed a range of local facilities like mosques, specialised groceries, take-away, cloth – shops and charities, providing them culturally relevant support and spaces for networking.

Various reasons for this clustering have been provided which include fear of racism, stigmatization, victims of crime among the external and convenience, social support, cultural practices among the internal factors (Lewis, 1994; Shah, 1998; Abbas, 2005). With its pre-1920 terraced houses and a high concentration of people of minority ethnic origin, Forest Fields is a well-known multi-cultural area situated northwest of Nottingham city centre. To the north, the area houses numerous small-scale industrial units, which are mostly derelict now. This area is known as New Basford. From the east the wealthy suburbs of Mapperley Park overlook Forest Fields, and from the West the area has extended into Aspley, which is mixed neighborhood housing with a large council estate and some affluent streets with detached properties and gardens. Most people of ethnic minority origin live in these areas of Nottingham city, making inner city Nottingham one of the most multi-ethnic areas, having dozens of mosques, Hindu temples and Gurdwara's, besides many churches and synagogues. Dr. Deborah Philips (1998) asserts that some members of the 'Muslim population are trapped in poor areas by their economic circumstances' and that moving away from these clusters is not seen an 'attractive alternative'. This is true in inner city Nottingham as 'clustering' is facilitated by 'positive community links, traditions and a sense of ethnic identity'. The fear of racial harassment and isolation adds to this clustering (Philips, 1998:5). Over a period of time, Forest Fields has become the hub of the South Asian, especially Mirpuri community, in Nottingham. When the author first arrived in Nottingham in the autumn of 1997, he found it like a town in South Asia. There were young boys walking in lines towards the mosques with skullcaps and clutching Qurans to their tiny chests. The aromas and colours of South Asian life were all over the place.

Many scholars have highlighted the relationship between place, social status and poverty (Levitas, 1998; Hardill et al., 2001). There are many deprived urban areas which house some of the most disadvantaged communities in the UK. The link between social conditions and geographic situation often results in the negative stereotyping of areas and people who live in these areas. Nottingham, characterized by high population density, also has image problem:

> *The area suffers from a poor reputation, although the main shopping road is not unduly run down. There also seems to be a strong sense of community, helping out, lift-giving etc. However people do not want to move there, businesses do not want to be based there and employers do not want to employ people from there. There have apparently been previous attempts at regeneration initiatives within the area.*

The 2001 Census was the first to contain a question on religion. The question was optional and in Nottingham city around 9.8% chose not to answer it. The number of people who classed themselves as Christian was 57.7 per cent, although this was significantly lower than the England fig. (71.7 per cent). Muslim (4.6 per cent) and Sikh (1.2 per cent) were the next most popular responses. About 24.8 per cent said they had no religion, which was much higher than the England fig. (4.6 per cent). The Muslim population of the UK comprising mostly Pakistanis (which includes Mirpuris), has a younger age profile, and almost half of them are born and brought up in the UK (ONS, 2001). While the majority of the Mirpuri community in Nottingham lives in Hyson Green, Radford and Basford area with the highest concentration in the Forest Fields area, some members of this community have now moved to Aspley, Wollaton, Mapperley and other richer areas of the city. But Forest Fields, with its mosques, special food shops, bookshops, boutiques and restaurants, has remained the focal point for the Mirpuri social and cultural life. Moreover, the extended family structure of this community means that people gravitate back, as the second and third generation Mirpuris who move out of the area often visit their parents and grandparents who prefer to live a gregarious life in the inner city.

A number of studies on the relation between religiosity and health have revealed a consistent link between the two (Levin, 1996). Within the Muslim population in the UK, the role of the mosque as a social and cultural reference is valued by Muslims. The institution of the mosque is also used by service providers to reach out to the members of the Muslim community. Islam highlights the importance of good health overtly and reminds every Muslims to look after their health and well-being as part of their religious duty. Islam views health as a state of complete physical, mental and social wellbeing. The Quran repeatedly emphasizes the importance of health with guidelines on healthy living, cleanliness and physical exercise, prohibition from intoxication and advice on food and nutrition (Quran 2:168, 5:90, 20:80, 55:7–9).

Although Islam clearly highlights the role of health and wellbeing in a just and equitable society, not much research has been undertaken to study the relationship between Islam and health behaviour. The first major effort to recognise the role of Islam in Health was the World Health Organisations' consultation on Islamic lifestyles and their impact on health development which took place in Amman in 1996 (Copy of the declaration is attached as Appendix E). The paper on recommendations of this consultation, known as Amman Declaration, identified more than 50 aspects of health, including nutrition, food safety, personal and community hygiene, waste disposal, sexual relationships, breast-feeding and child care, mental health, alcohol consumption and substance abuse, on which the Islamic teachings could offer guidance. There are over 1000 purpose-built and makeshift mosques in the UK, and many of these mosques are not active in the social and cultural life of the communities they serve. However, some big mosques offer people services in issues related to culture and faith but these Mosques have now extended their role in delivering culturally sensitive interventions in health, education and employment. Besides the mosques, Muslim health professionals, including doctors have set up national organisations and institutions in the UK to educate members of the Muslim community on health issues. The Muslim Health Network (MHN) was established to play a principal role in promoting, preserving, and protecting health amongst the Muslim communities in the UK. The aim of the network is to improve the standard of health and wellbeing within the community through information, support, news, advice, events and the promotion of general health issues. Similarly, the Muslim Doctors and Dentists Association (MDDA) provide consultation and support to mosques and other institutions to promote healthy living among the Muslim communities in the UK. While faith based institutions have been on rise, the state institutions have not been able to engage with such institutions to reach out to the communities.

One of the failures of social policy in the UK is seen to be its disproportionate focus on the social while overlooking the cultural and political aspects. The official discourse of social exclusion/inclusion does not engage with the knowledge and experience of marginalized people. The practice of health promotion is one clear example of the lack of appreciation of the cultural practices of people in fighting inequalities in health. Health promotion is largely seen to be influenced by the Ottawa Charter for Health Promotion endorsed by the WHO, 1986. This charter has come under increasing criticism for reflecting a Western, post-Cartesian value system (Davies & MacDonald, 1998). However, some scholars and practitioners now see the concept of health promotion as a practice influenced by faith and culture, and argue that health awareness is supported by Quranic texts. These scholars conceptualise an alternative vision of health promotion informed by the Islamic value system (Leeuw & Hussein, 1999). The Health Education Awareness Project, which was the highlight of Radio Ramzan's broadcast in 1999–2000, brought all these debates into focus by demonstrating the need to develop a contextual approach in addressing inequalities in health that recognizes the agency of culture and faith.

The Birth of Radio Ramzan in Nottingham

Though there were a number of mosques and religious centres in Nottingham, it was the Karimia Mosque which operated from a local Mosque in Forest Fields, a neighbourhood of predominantly South Asian community that was a popular hub for religious, social and cultural activities in inner city area. The Mosque applied for a license in first time in 1997 to run a community radio station on restricted service during the month of Ramadan, the month of Fasting in Islamic calendar. The license was awarded, and Radio Ramzan started broadcasting in and around Nottingham City on the 29th of December 1997 on 97.5 FM. It became the fourth such station to be awarded a license to broadcast during the month of Ramadan in the UK under the Restricted Service License (RSL) scheme run by the Radio Authority (now Ofcom). On behalf of the Muslim community, Karimia Mosque obtained the license, and owing to its to its central position among Nottingham's Barailve Muslim population, it mobilised the human and material resources to support this project. The station was established on Radford Road in Forest Field, the heart of the Mirpuri community in Nottingham, and soon different voices and points of views could be heard on this radio station. Muslim communities in Nottingham. Being a community radio using a variety of South Asian languages especially Mirpuri/Punjabi, the station generated a fair amount of interest in Nottingham, particularly among the Mirpuri population. Since Muslims have an obligation to fast, pray and give charity during this month, the Radio helped members of the community to focus on more communal issues and highlight their cultural practices. The fact that people could hear Adhan (call for prayers) in their homes, cars, shops and businesses five times a day added a new cultural dimension to the organization of daily life.

As the station was allowed under restricted service license, the Karimia Mosque, the parent organization took the initiative of organising a community wide consultation with the main objectives of seeking public participation in running a community-wide radio station, explore the topics, treatments and approaches in debating issues pertinent to the community, and to find resources through avenues for partnerships, sponsorships and donations for the running of this station.

This was perhaps the first meeting in Nottingham among the Muslim groups, which was very well attended by people from various walks of life. Most of the community organizations, business people, councilors and representatives from various other mosques attended. After deliberation for over two hours, it was decided to make the radio station open and to all, a community-wide organising committee, including members from the women organization, should facilitate representation of all shades of opinion. The deliberations the meeting clearly stated that besides celebrating the month of Ramadan, the radio should raise social, political and economic issues that impact the local communities in Nottingham. The disaffection of young people from the community was highlighted during the meeting and their involvement in running this community venture was sought. To represent view, aspirations and issues faced by the groups within the Muslim community, it was also decided to use a combination of languages including English, Mirpuri and Urdu, Bengali, Gujarati and Pashto languages. The public meeting also suggested that the Radio station shoud be used for raising funds for charity causes. A constitution for the station was adopted and four committees to look after the programming, advertising, technical side and public relations for the radio station were constituted. After all these discussions and preparations, Radio Ramzan became a reality when the signature tune of this station on 97.5 FM was played followed by the Fajar Adan (call for morning prayers) on Monday the 29th of December, 1997. It was the first day of fasting and people were glued to their radio sets. Weeks of publicity, especially the announcements in local mosques and the word of mouth generated a huge interest. The author was with a group of volunteers listening to the signature tune, and he could see joy on the faces of everyone in the studio and instantly phones started to ring.

The radio station added significance to this special month of Ramadan as it broadcasts daily five times Adhan (calls to prayer). These timings are crucial to determine the beginning and end of fasting. This focused the attention of whole Muslim community on the radio, so it was not just in the background to fill the space, but a critical factor in time, providing a social context to the spiritual life. In a local situation the radio helped to forge that communal feeling by organizing communal activities and socially re-organises the community by providing locally relevant information. Certain differences within the community are overcome while others are acknowledged. One example of this negotiation is the programme schedule of Radio Ramzan, which reflects a variety of languages (Urdu, Arabic, Mirpuri, Punjabi, Bengali, Gujarati and English) and formats to suit various ethnic and sub-ethnic groups within the construct of Muslim community

The radio station, located within the heart of the Mirpuri community in the Forest Fields/ Hyson Green area, had made it part of the community calendar in Nottingham. Hence the expectations of the 1999–2000 Radio Ramzan from its listeners were high. There was already a section of the community who wanted a permanent station, but there were others who opposed this idea. The last two Radio Ramzan had raised the profile of the Karimia Mosque and it had attained the distinction of working on social and economic issues pertinent to the community. This experience helped Karimia to network with the Police, Housing, Health and Leisure Departments, along with the local council officials and politicians flocked to the radio. Broadcasting through this medium was proving a cost-effective way to reach out to the 'hard to reach' groups. Radio Ramzan also gave the legitimacy to the information provided due to its association with the Karimia Mosque and the fact the broadcasting was taking place in the month of Ramadan.

It was not just content but the context which was critical in this process of communication. While education and employment remained the focus of the previous two Radio Ramzans, the third radio series was dedicated to the issues around the health of minority ethnic groups, especially that of Mirpuri community in Nottingham. In association with the Specialist Health Promotion Service of Nottingham Health Authority, Karimia Mosque developed a comprehensive health education project using Radio Ramzan as a vehicle to reach out to the community and seek their participation in developing culturally sensitive and socially relevant strategies to fight inequalities in health. The role of voluntary organisations, including community groups, in supporting the people belonging to minority groups in education, health, housing, immigration issues and employment is well established within the discourse of community development (Mayo & Craig, 1995). The voluntary sector is known to facilitate involvement of local people in community affairs (Farnell et al., 2003).

This partnership approach between public and voluntary sector has become part of a new discourse in which the concepts of community mobilization and local participation are sought to reduce health inequalities and promote good health among marginalised groups. Supported by many surveys and research findings, the participatory approach in health education and delivery is highlighted in various health policy documents (Acheson, 1998; Department of Health, 1999; Social Exclusion Unit, 2000). This approach is also present in various international declarations supported by World Health Organisation (WHO) including Alma Ata Declaration (1978), the Ottawa Charter (1986), Amman Declaration (1996) and Jakarta Declaration (1997). However, the populist paradigm of participation has come under attack for its technical, theoretical, political and conceptual limitations. There is a range of critiques available about the populist participation approach (Bastian & Bastian, 1996; Nelson & Wright, 1995). Although there are critics of this approach who question the rhetorical use of participation and demand clarification on terms, mechanism and conditions of partnerships and alliances (Cooke & Kothari, 2003), the approach of involving victims of inequality to fight inequality does make sense when participation is on the terms of victims.

As discussed in Chap. 5, the inequalities in health are a combination of social, economic and political issues, and one way to deal with them is to empower people so that they understand the causes and consequences of this inequality. Empowerment is possible only when people participate or when their involvement is facilitated rather than enforced or managed. Looking at the literature on the participatory approaches in dealing with health inequalities, three major models emerge; Management approach to Participation, Social Capital approach to Participation and Empowerment approach to Participation. Traditionally, the community politics are ridden with divisions and differences; however, it does show tactical and strategic unity on issues of commonality through shared commitments and cooperation bringing people together. The month of Ramadan proved a common factor for various groups to support it and show an act of solidarity, but this unity did not work on every issue. As we will find out later in detail in this chapter, an open debate on the subject of sighting of the Moon led to a very awkward situation, and the live discussion on the radio had to be cut off in order to pacify the public.

While differences were seen more on philosophical and doctrinal issues among various groups, ordinary listeners were not that much bothered about the big issues.

They were finding radio very useful but would not like differences to be exposed in public. Another positive aspects of this radio station was the enthusiasm and entrepreneurial flair of its, mostly young, volunteers. This passion kept the things moving even with limited resources and expertise. The voluntary sector with limited capacity and resources depends on volunteers and Radio Ramzan had no dearth of such volunteers. FY manned telephones in early mornings before he went to college. He said he loved the place: *We discuss Islam, politics and so on so freely without any fear. Tell me where is this possible? Even in Pakistan you cannot talk about all these things. You know what I mean?*

KM who lived in Meadows area of the city, heard the radio accidentally while driving one day in the city, and rang to offer help in the programme production. Within a week, he had his own show in which he interviewed young entrepreneurs from the community. He said:

> *It all happened accidentally. I was waiting to pick up my kids from the school. While waiting, I was pressing the frequency button on my car radio when I heard the Adan. I removed finger from the button and the dial was read 97.5 FM Radio Ramzan. It was unbelievable! A Muslim radio in Nottingham!! I kept it on, collected my kids from the school and kept listening. It got more and more interesting. There was a Qawali (traditional Sufi singing style from South Asia, popularized by Pakistani singers) followed by a commercial break.... they were selling all familiar things...Chicken Tikka, vegetables, cheap air tickets and they were asking for charity for people in Kashmir and Afghanistan. The commercial break was followed a discussion on race. For the first time I felt engaged with something, and I wanted to be part of this. Reaching home, I asked my wife to put the radio on 97.5. It was coming closer to Magrib time (time to open fast) and everyone in the family was now listening. Later in the evening I rang and asked if I could help. I was told to come the next day.*

However, community being a very complex construct of competing power relations exhibits different levels and intensities of these relation as power over, power on and power to becomes critically important. The running of the radio station exposed certain power relations, which normally remain invisible. The power to say things or the concept of 'voice', is a political construct, and the condition of not having a is seen as powerlessness. This concept of empowerment was put in practice, when the radio provided a platform for various people to come forward, organize themselves and support younger members of the community to achieve better in education. Poor performance in education is a perennial issues within Mirpuri community in the UK, especially those who in the post industrial deprived inner city areas. The 'Empowerment through Education' project/campaign was started on the station to attract teachers from the community to help local children in afterschool clubs and Sunday classes. The project raised enough interest through discussions, debates and phone-ins and it encouraged a number of teachers and professionals from the community to come forward to run evening and weekend classes forin Maths and English at the local Karimia Mosque. Children from as far as Sneinton, Basford, Carlton, Wollaton and Beeston came to attend these classes. Encouraged by this response, Karimia Mosque approached the local regeneration budget and was able to get funding for three years from the Single Regeneration Budget (SRB) to support these classes. As class sizes increased, Karimia approached Forest School The school also benefited from this project, as most of the children who attend these classes were students of this school. The children were getting one-to one support in a culturally relevant environment. A parent, HI, whose children benefited from this project said:

> *Everyone is a winner from this project. Karimia gets more members, children get help in Math and English, Forest Schools get support for its pupils and parents can keep children off the streets. This project was made possible when people made a lot noise that our kids are not doing well in education.*

A log of the phone calls received by the station showed 80 per cent of the calls came from these areas of the city. It can be argued that the very presence of Radio Ramzan in the community generated responses and debates at a larger level by opening up a space wherein people negotiate and align strategically on a common ground. During the month of Ramadan, this strategy becomes more important for Muslims due to the heightened consciousness about the 'community' which is reinforced time and again during this month through sermons, festivities and the ritual of fasting. Radio Ramzan mirrors this feeling on a community-wide platform. While religion remains main focus of this radio, it helps to blend the social, economic, political and spiritual of life. Through this process the community becomes a dynamic construct that creates solidarities across divisions and differences.

McQuail (1994) has highlighted the role of the horizontal patterns of such democratic communication necessary for social action. But it will be naive to think that this radio station can overcome all the social, political, cultural and economic disadvantages the Mirpuri community faces. Similarly, to assume that Radio Ramzan can represent all the shades of Muslim communities will not be only impractical but also misleading. The differences and divisions within the Muslim groups are a result of historical and doctrinal perspectives that cannot be resolved on a radio show. Although Radio Ramzan could be heard in the whole of Nottingham's urban areas and in some outskirts as well, its loyal audience lives in Forest Fields, Radford, Basford, Hyson Green, Lenton, Sneinton and Basford. These are the areas with the highest concentration of Muslims.

Health Inequalities at the Local Level

Despite representing a large proportion of the UK minority ethnic population, health statistics comparing people of South Asian origin with the general population highlight significant health inequalities. Pakistani (mostly Mirpuri) and Bangladeshi (mostly Syelhetti) people, predominantly Muslim, have rates of cardiovascular disease 60 per cent to 70 per cent higher than men in the general population. Similarly, the prevalence of Diabetes, Obesity and the rate of premature deaths due to Coronary heart disease are significantly higher among these people than the rest of the population. These figures, however, need to be taken with caution as disparities occur between people of various origins and between men and women among the South Asian population. Whatever may be the variables and differences with various

South Asian communities, one thing is clear that these groups suffer from significant health inequalities, which also correspond with the levels of material deprivation these communities face. Social and material conditions are considered to have a direct impact on the health of people, and Mirpuri communities have been identified as suffering 50 per cent higher rates of Coronary heart disease than other comparative ethnic groups and five times the risk of developing Diabetes (Nazroo, 1997). It will be, however, simplistic to collapse ethnicity and poverty into poor health. Issues like racism, culture, ethnic identity and factors shaping peoples' participation are also seen as valid factors in determining the health of people and communities (Nazroo, 1998; Smaje, 1996; Williams et al., 1997).

Chapter 5 of this thesis explores the issues around health inequalities like racialisation of health, healthism and managerialism in health services. Part of the problem is that the discourse of healthism depends on the Western medical model of health which sees well-being as a state of the body without disease. This clinical understanding of health ignores or dismisses the role of cultural practices and beliefs of people in improving their health and feeling well while there is an established correlation between poverty, ethnicity and poorer health (Wilkinson, 1996; Nazroo, 2000). In Nottingham itself, many policy, structural and procedural issues have been argued to contribute to the health service's inadequacy in dealing with the health needs of minority ethnic groups, especially, the Mirpuri community which is the largest ethnic group in Nottingham (Nerwal, 1997)

A detailed survey to explore ways of reaching this hard-to-reach group and addressing the issues of health inequality faced by the Mirpuri community was undertaken by the Health Education Authority in association with the Nottingham Education Authority, Nottingham Community Trust and Nottingham Borough and the County Councils as a national-local partnership. This three year survey, which started in 1997, is seen as one of the most comprehensive action research projects to explore the issues of access, reach and inequality in health in Forest Fields, Lenton, Radford and Trent – four wards of Nottingham city. The survey, among other underlying issues, explored the fact that health services traditionally fail to deal adequately with the health needs of ethnic minorities and to reduce their inequitable access to health and related services. The survey acknowledged the fact that attempts to redress this imbalance have most often taken the form of project-based initiatives, and at the end of the projects there is little evidence to show that the resultant service implications become funded through the primary commissioning and planning processes of agencies.

The research which forms the foundation of health promotion initiatives in Nottingham recommended that instead of ghettoising services by creating specialised services for non-white population, positive action should be taken to mainstream the services for ethnic minorities. The report suggested training mainstream service providers about the cultural and social issues of minority groups and sensitising them to the needs and fears of this group. The report also pointed out those short-term, ad hoc and token gestures by Health services worsen the health inequalities and suggested an ongoing sustained policy and better means of communication and raising awareness through multi-agency information delivery which could empower those who are marginalized to take control of their health. One of the striking features of this report was the recommendation of using action research as both a delivery and evaluation tool in addressing inequalities.

A Health Needs Assessment (HNA) carried out by the Nottingham Health Authority in 1996 provided some basic information on the nature, extent and causes of health inequality related to ethnicity in Nottingham. Harjinder Nerwal, who worked as a social worker on black and minority ethnic health issues, found that cultural beliefs and language were the major barriers for people of minority origin to access services, and that lack of cultural sensitivity by the service providers added to the helplessness of these people. The report (Nerwal, 1997) specifically pointed out the lack or reluctance of providing information on specific and general services, including the availability of female doctors, facilities for male circumcision. Prejudice towards non-English speaking people and the lack of recreational facilities, community transport, along with poor housing, and the isolation within which older members of this community, especially women, lived were also highlighted in this report. The report suggested that people of minority ethnic origin should be empowered in terms of how services should be provided, keeping in view their social needs and cultural sensitivities. The report recommended that communication was crucial in such empowerment and information should be available in verbal and written formats about health issues within the community setting, via Asian health professionals, workshops, seminars, and Asian Radio Programmes as well as leaflets and posters (Nerwal, 1997, p. 46).

Health Education Awareness Project (HEAP)

As part of its third broadcast season in December 1999, Radio Ramzan buoyant with its popularity among the local Muslim community in Nottingham, developed a multi-agency 'Health Education Awareness Project' (HEAP) approach to address health inequalities within the living experiences of its audience. The HEAP, which chronicled a month-long health education campaign, engaged social aspects of life with the spiritual to develop a unique health promotion programme in which members of the Muslim communities enter into debates and discussions about situation to develop initiatives for empowerment through critical reflection and collective action. The project focused on the most pertinent health problems within this community which include Coronary heart diseases, Diabetes and Obesity, Mental Health, Smoking, Sexual health etc. in a unique partnership between public and voluntary sector to mobilize community and increase their participation in the campaign.

The process of conceiving and delivering the HEAP project involved developing strategies to bridge the gulf between theory and practice. While we had the broad principles of participation and empowerment guiding us, it was the actual practice of situating these principles within the faith, culture and experiences of marginalized people that made the process meaningful. Developing, practicing and recording this project revealed a number of processes and generated many issues concerning the use of community-based media in fighting inequalities.

The project was basically a partnership project between the City Central Primary Care Trust (PCT) in Nottingham and the Karimia Mosque. While Dr. MH was the main person from the Karimia, RM, then Chief Executive of the City Central PC T represented the NHS in the project. This month-long intensive health education campaign brought together local people, health professionals, community workers, religious leaders, volunteers and statutory organizations to find a common ground to fight inequalities in health. This was first such project where the victims of inequalities would enter into a discursive space with the policy makers and practitioners to address issues from their own experiences and cultural context. In this process, the legitimization of subjectivity becomes epistemologically and methodologically critical, as marginalized voices and experiences enter into the research.

The objectives of the HEAP project included:

- Generate and share knowledge from the experiences of health from participants, which can be used as guidance for change to promote health education and mobilization for culturally relevant action.
- Develop a contextual approach in addressing some of the pertinent health issues among the Mirpuri community by acknowledging and adopting the cultural practices prevalent in this community.
- Facilitate the participation of marginalized people in local health initiatives so that they can take a more pro-active part in looking after their health and the health of others in the community.
- Raise awareness about health services in general and about rights and responsibilities of people in particular.

As the third year of Radio Ramzan approached, the Primary Care Trust (PCT) City Central – a city focused health initiative of the National Health Service (NHS)-was introduced to address the health inequalities in the area. The role of the PCT to improve health through developing partnerships with the local community presented a great opportunity for the Karimia Mosque. The PCT covering the geographical area within which the Karimia Mosque was based was City Central. When the PCT City Central was approached to formalize a partnership they were not only very keen but excited to work with the Karimia.

RM, then Chief Executive of the City Central PCT, sums up the keenness of the National Health Service (NHS) to work with the Karimia on this health education project using the unique medium of Radio Ramzan: There was a huge advantage to us in having a strong partnership with Karimia Mosque. The interpretation of our health messages within an Islamic perspective added authority to what we were saying and increased the chances that listeners would take notice of what was being said. The partnership with Karimia Mosque also helped us to raise sensitive issues such as sexual health and domestic violence within an Islamic framework (RM, 2001). The subsequent project proposal which developed fitted in with the PCT City Central's objectives and priority area and offered an opportunity for the NHS to develop a stronger community partnership and develop the potential capacity building opportunities.

From the Karimia point of view, this was an opportunity to address the health issues and make the mosque more meaningful to the social realities of local Muslim population. This was also an opportunity to engage with service providers and give them first insight into cultural practices of people they ought to service. Dr. MH, the Imam of the Karimia Mosque, and the architect of faith based social intervention in Nottingham, said:

> *Historically, mosque has played a pivotal role in Muslim societies. But due to the Western mind set, spirituality has been reduced to a private thing. Karimia is trying to bring Mosque back to the forefront of the public life and use this important resource in developing Muslim communities. Projects like HEAP help us to bring service providers and users together to make interventions meaningful for those who need the services most. It helps government and other agencies to understand the cultural context of the people who they are trying to engage with. Health projects like HEAP benefit us all.* (Based on interview with MH. Jan, 2000)

The PCT and Karimia made a joint steering group to develop the HEAP project. While SK, a local health practitioner to lead the project, the committee had the following members:

- RM, City Central PCT
- MSF, a local Imam
- Dr. ZK, GP at Mary Potters health centre
- SW, NHS Direct
- RS, a youth worker
- TK, local teacher

The committee met twice and deliberated on the topics, structure and delivery of the HEAP project. The following topics were identified to as appropriate for the Radio shows:

- Introductory show- Health Inequalities
- Coronary Heart Disease and Diabetes
- Stroke and Physical Activity
- Smoking cessation
- Diet and Nutrition
- Asthma
- Accident Prevention
- Sexual Health
- Mental Health
- Thalassemia
- Domestic Violence

(A copy of the HEAP schedule is enclosed as Appendix G)

The following additions were made while the project was running, due to requests from various agencies and organisations to become part of the HEAP project:

- The Interpretation Service
- The Radford Visiting Scheme
- The African Caribbean Asian Forum.

Based on the most common health issues prevelant in this community, the HEAP project was structured around following tangible outcomes:

- Production and broadcast of 12, one hour-long interactive, radio shows on various health issues pertinent to minority ethnic groups.
- Production of Public Service Announcements (PSA) of 60 seconds duration in Mirpuri, Urdu, Bengali (Syelhetti) and English. These PSA to be played on the hourly basis round the clock during the month of Ramadan.
- A competition on health issues to keep the community involved with the project. A seminar at the end of the project to get feedback from public and evaluate the success of the HEAP.
- My own recollection and reflection (based on field notes).
- Documentary evidence such as policy documents, publicity material, minutes of meetings, agendas, reports, letters, emails, phone calls.
- Feedback from open days and comments on evaluation forms.
- Interviews with 12 people involved in the running of the HEAP project.

The topics selected for discussion reflected both national and local policy, priorities and plans including the Health Improvement Programme and Health Action Zone. The topics also reflected pertinent issues concerning the Mirpuri/Pakistani and Bangladeshi communities. While a panel of professionals, local people and a religious leader provided advice on the various aspects of this project, it was the Mirpuri-speaking health practitioner SK who worked for the Specialist Health Promotions Scheme of the Nottingham Health Authority who proved a real asset for this project.

RR is a British born second generation Mirpuri whose parents had migrated to the UK in the 1960's. She has lived all her life in Nottingham and understood the social, cultural and political aspects of ethnic minority life in Nottingham very well. She is part of an effective community worker network which proved very beneficial to the HEAP project. Her greatest asset was the understanding of the health issues, and she is very 'political' about the issues around health inequalities.

The author worked closely with her to develop this project. While her background, knowledge of the subject, an impressive contact list and her position in the community were key factors that determined the course of HEAP project, my background in media, association with Karimia Mosque and my role as coordinator of Radio Ramzan helped to put things together and deliver it within a tight schedule and budget. We both shared the political views and passion that argued for validation of marginalised perspectives and we both were very vocal and active in promoting them. Reflecting on why she chose to develop a health project this way, she said:

> *Radio Ramzan was different. It was not the mainstream media...you know what I mean. It was for people who would not normally listen to the BBC or Trent FM. Radio Ramzan would give a different point of view, and everyone wanted to hear that. My favourite was the*

late night show...It was a fantastic current affairs prog and talked about today's issues and the challenges community faced. And all these issue whether social, political or economic are inter-related and have an impact on health. So you cannot put health in that medical box...it is all connected. Radio Ramzan helped to look at health as a whole and not just from the clinical point of view. This is important for a community that is disadvantaged and faces inequalities in health. I remember some of the issues touched in the HEAP programmes were picked up by other programmes and there was continuing debate on the following day. In fact the debates were not confined to radio only. As a community worker I know how these discussions cascaded down. The month of Ramadan added values to these debates. The shows on sex education, mental health and smoking had a better reception as the Karimia Mosque gave the health education campaign the much need cultural legitimacy and social proximity. (RR, 2000, excerpts from a recorded interview)

SK provided the matrix for the HEAP project and also identified resource persons and wrote the scripts for the shows. The author fronted this project by hosting the radio show and working with a team of volunteers who would be at the reception, do the technical tasks and take phone calls during the show. This small team of people knew each other and gelled together well. The author had first seen JM, the receptionist, in the mosque coming regularly for prayers. He later joined the Karimia Sunday school and played cricket with local lads. JM is the nephew of a member of the management committee member of Karimia Mosque. His uncle AM was the main person who looked after the technical side of the radio. AM worked as a network engineer at a computer company in Derby and was a regular attendee at the Karimia Mosque. AM and JM belonged to the local Mistaree Biradari and were very well connected in the community.

Their presence at the radio station attracted lot more young people, and in the afternoon and evenings, particularly at the time of Magrib (dusk) Radio Ramzan would be buzzing with activity. These young men were keen to do voice-overs, find music and tidy up the place. Having this commitment and ownership of the Radio was crucial in delivering the HEAP project which relied heavily on volunteers in outreach, production, delivery and evaluation of this health education programme on Radio Ramzan. While the Karimia and Radio Ramzan were lacking capacity and financial resources, though it had dependable human resources in terms of volunteers who would make things happen. The centrality of the Karimia Mosque in the social life of the local Mirpuri population kept these volunteers focused, and there was an incentive of 'creating our own media'.

This sense of achievement was more intense among the younger generation of Mirpuri people, born and brought up in the UK; as JM put it:

Although I'm into reggae and stuff like that but at the end of the day I cannot be what I'm not. Do you see what I mean? I'm a Mirpuri...speak Mirpuri and love Desi life style. But the problem is we do not have a voice, we are seen as outsiders though I was born here and my mates are Gora (white). Radio Ramzan may not be the best thing but at least something we can own and make noise about.

Melkote and Steeve (2001), mapping the debates on empowerment led perspectives, argue that the cultural practices of people are detrimental for the success of community-based projects. They highlight, within the context of developing countries, the role of religious organisation and motivation in the fight against discrimination' and disadvantage (2001: 293). From above comments it is clear that reference to religion is not divorced from the social aspects of life. The HEAP project was conceived and delivered within this context.

The First Show

In the first live radio, Dr. MH of Imam Of Karimia Mosque, RM, City Central PCT Chief executive, HT NHS Direct Communication and training manager, Dr. ZK Local General practitioner, Ms. RR, NHS bilingual, worker raised curtain on the month long, multi-agency Health awareness project. The show adopted a multi-language approach using Mirpuri, English and Urdu languages. RR translated and summed up from English into Mirpuri while the rest of the panelists switched between Urdu, Mirpuri and English. Dr. ZK, a Mirpuri himself, spoke in Mirpuri and gave valuable insights into the health issues, peoples' expectations and his constraints as a General Practitioner working for a local health centre.

On a question about his experiences of being a Mirpuri doctor in an area with a large number of Mirpuri people Dr. ZK said:

> *There are many people from our community who want to spend bit more time with me and talk about the issues which are not necessarily about health but have a direct impact on their well-being. The isolation, family problems, cultural issues etc.but I cannot. I wish I had time to do that. We are not necessarily addressing the core context, but we take a very narrow view of illness. I cannot do more than prescribe a pill. No doubt there are provisions for referring people, but the culture these people come from does not operate this way. In their culture doctor is very important. The minute we refer them to someone else they have this feeling of being ignored and not given the best advice.* (Dr ZK on Radio Ramzan, December 1999)

RM:

> *This is the predicament. While NHS is trying its best to provide a culturally and socially appropriate service, the inadequacy of resources on one hand and expectations of service users on the other hand make it hard to strike a balance. I agree that health issues need to look at the context and develop a holistic approach, but we need to learn more and know more. The HEAP is an ideal platform to exchange ideas.*

Dr. MH

> *This is responsibility of NHS to offer appropriate services for people of various cultural backgrounds and give them a say in the running of services for them. So far we have only seen tokenism. Things can only improve when there are long term partnerships with community groups who should be used in the delivery of services rather than being used or the sake of partnerships.*

Dr. ZK intervened:

> *This is a two-way process. People also have to come forward and make their views and comments heard. Community groups and Mosques like Karimia can play an important role in initiating a dialogue between service providers and users. It is not just health but in every aspect, places like Mosques are crucial. Having said that there are issues around women's*

participation. Mosques still remain predominantly male dominated, and we have to be imaginative to get women involved in these debates and issues.

A caller who did not want to be identified:

In our society, unfortunately, everything is decided by men even the doctor and health service. Women have many problems and going to doctor sometimes is not helpful. Women need to be culturally more appropriate places and venues where they can access the services. I'm obese, and suffering from Diabetes, I cannot go for swimming and gym in mixed places ...what I'm trying to say is we need such facilities within our community.

RM responds:

We do understand the sensitivities around women's issues, especially among the women of South Asian origin. We are providing language and interpretation service to address these issues but obviously we need to do more. Maybe the community will have to come forward and work with other agencies to provide services which can help people like this caller....

Dr. MH of Karimia:

As an Imam I understand the problems faced by our community. The women need service provisions that look at the sensitivities of being a Mirpuri woman. That is why it will be appropriate for the government to develop Mosques as places where such services can be provided. At the Karimia, we have made some progress in this regard. (Discussion on Live Radio)

Reflecting on the whole debate, it was felt that neither the health centre in a mosque nor having a translator at the mainstream health centre can solve the issues raised by the caller. The caller, by raising the important issue of patriarchy within the Mirpuri community, was also offering a solution by asking for community-based provisions for staying healthy. The answers and assurances from the service providers were within the discourse of 'Healthism' where the problem is seen to be at the receiving end. The service of NHS Direct is not very relevant here. Even if a woman wants to go to their drop-in centre, she needs permission to get out of the house, and in many cases does not drive herself, and need a transport. Above all, the real or perceived fear of racism makes it harder for such women to venture out of their houses and access mainstream services. Unfamiliarity with procedural matters while accessing such services makes things even harder.

Dr. MH's assertion that mosque can fill the gap where service providers cannot reach is not a complete solution. Mosques, especially in the UK, remain a male phenomenon. Very few mosques have provisions for women, and the women who find it hard to access services at mainstream centres will be no more comfortable with using such services at mosques. My concerns were echoed by RR who, herself being a Mirpuri woman, understands these issues very well. However, we agreed that an hour-long radio programme is no way near to offering solutions to the complex problem of health inequality, but the fact that these issues were being discussed on a community wide platform is in itself an achievement. It was interesting to see those who hold bureaucratic, professional and religious power being questioned by those who these people exercise power over.

The power, temporarily though, was shifting from these powerful persons to less powerful listeners of radio who were in a position to decide what and what not to listen to and at the same time ask difficult questions making the panel answerable. Post-structuralism theory helps to understand the circularity of power relations in the production of subjectivities (Hollway, 1984). Thus, the ways and means through which particular groups are marginalized can be uncovered by delving into the hierarchies of power that construct our realities (Kamler et al., 1994). This way Foucault provides a tool which can explain how power is exercised through discourse and how resistance is possible against this exercise.

Generally, within the health services, the authoritative power is magnified and exercised through offices, receptions, uniforms, appointments and translations. It is the territory – the office, the health centre- which makes one think of being in a powerless situation. Being ill and weak makes things even worse. Through the discourse of 'healthism' of which traditional health promotion is a big part, subjects are produced which then go through self-regulation. Foucault explains that the modern subject is the creation of 'power' and 'self'. He sees power as directing the conduct of others who through self-surveillance and normalization, become objects of control (Foucault, 1979). Foucault's metaphor of the 'Panopticon' helps to understand this power/knowledge dynamic. Radio Ramzan disturbs this dynamic as it takes the powerful out of their comfort zones and puts them in fuzzy, messy and real situations where the whole theory of 'responsibilisation' or acting in a certain way becomes irrelevant as people foreground their own worldviews and ways of life. In a way, the space offered by Radio Ramzan enables a counter- discourse where people were using a reference to their faith, culture and their experiences help them change the power dynamics, temporarily.

The second Radio show on the 10th of December, 1999 had the theme of Coronary heart diseases (CHD) a common ailment among the people of South Asian origin.

Coronary Heart Diseases

Coronary heart disease (CHD) is the UK's single biggest killer. More than 110,000 people die of heart problems each year. Around 41,000 of these deaths are premature, and most of the premature deaths due to CHD are thought to be among the people of South Asian origin. The death rate is 46 per cent higher for men and 51 per cent higher for women (BHF, 2000). While it is not completely known why South Asians suffer more from heart disease than other groups, several explanations have been suggested, like genetic susceptibilities, metabolic disorders associated with insulin resistance, and general obesity. Besides this medical explanation, it is also suggested that the disadvantaged socio-economic position of South Asians, especially people of Mirpuri and Bangladeshi origin, may be also contributing to the higher rates of CHD among these people. This is also linked to higher rates of smoking, low rates of exercise and a diet high in fat and low in fruit and vegetables. One striking findings that all these ailments and conditions tend to be diagnosed at a more advanced stage of disease among the people of South Asian origin and the survival rates seem to be poor.

With this background and statistical evidence, the CHD debate was the priority of HEAP. In the second radio show, Dr. ZK was joined by another local general practitioner Dr. Packham and the Diabetes worker ST along with the Mirpuri bilingual worker Rashida. In the first part of the show, doctors explained the symptoms and consequences of heart problems especially CHD, in the latter part of the show Shaista discussed the necessary precautions in the lifestyle, especially food and need for physical exercise. The topic, having a higher relevance to our audience, proved very popular in terms of phone calls we had during the shows. While most of the callers were inquiring about their specific conditions, some questions raised wider issues around service provisions and the role of community in helping raise awareness about the problem. One of the callers, who did not want to be identified, spoke in English and questioned the sustainability of a project like HEAP:

> *We are sick of having these one off events...which help no one. There has to be a long term planning of helping people on a long terms basis. I have been living with this problem for nearly 10 years now, and I know what the cause of this problem is. What is the government doing to address the causes? Everybody looks at how to manage the problem and NHS...just to show on paper they are reaching out to minority people do things like this. Heart problem, obesity, sugar problem are common and have been there always...so where was NHS before. It is good to have radio shows like this but the question is what happens after the month of Ramadan. The diseases do not go away. In fact, we'll start eating like before and will be even worse.* (Radio Ramzan Listener who went on air to air his comments, December, 1999)

A very valid comment with which the doctors agreed and only Shaista reacted:

> *It is not completely true that there is no follow up. The Diabetes team goes to community centres...we have been to mosques and at times do home visits to help people but community should come forward and have something like, for example, Radio Ramzan to reinforce the message again and again.* (Live discussion on Radio, Dec. 2000)

Reflecting on this debate, SK was of the opinion that sustainability is only possible in a stable environment. She said that no doubt the health professionals are keen to develop a long term strategy to deal with inequalities but regretted the fact that too many changes within the NHS itself throw everything out of the window.

> *I would not say that commitment is not there...but I would say the constant change in health and in the public sector does not allow the sustainability...it does not allow to build on something which is good. When management structure changes, the priority changes and so does the funding and focus. We had too many changes in the Health Authority in last few years. There's no consistency.* (SK, Post programme discussion to reflect on the issues raised in the first show of HEAP on Radio Ramzan, Jan 2000)

The issue of sustainability is indispensable to health promotion, especially about those diseases which are linked to the lifestyle of people. CHD is believed to be caused by a number of risk factors, of which many can be influenced. Evidence suggested that modifiable lifestyle factors such as smoking, lack of physical activity and poor diet all contribute to the increased risk of CHD in South Asian groups. The British Heart Foundation (2000) suggests that in order to make the strategies focusing on these risk factors effective, information needs to reach to the right people and such strategies need to take into account the language and cultural barriers and be targeted appropriately. So the medium of Radio Ramzan perhaps is the appropriate means to reach to the people and raise awareness about the risk factors linked to CHD, but the question is when that community does not have resources or capacity to run long term health projects, how could these campaigns be sustained, and who should fund them?

Smoking and Substance Misuse

One of the major risk factors linked to cardiovascular disease and CHD is smoking, and this issue was discussed thoroughly in the third show under the HEAP programme on Radio Ramzan. In England alone, it is believed that about ten million people smoke– over one in four people. Stopping smoking is considered the single most important thing a smoker can do to avoid a heart attack. Overall, South Asian men continue to smoke more than the general population, although smoking levels vary widely between and within ethnic groups. About 42 per cent of Bangladeshi men are smokers compared with 27 per cent of men in the general population. (Joint Health Surveys Unit, 2001)

Being a common problem among Radio Ramzan listeners, the show was given a higher priority. The Karimia Mosque had invited smoking cessation workers and doctors to the mosque before Ramadan to help its members to give up smoking. Dr. MH was keen to use the medium of Radio Ramzan in this regard. During the month of Ramadan, members of the Muslim communities do not normally eat, drink or smoke during daylight hours. Ramadan thus gives the useful focus for raising awareness among people about the risks associated with smoking and how the habit can be given up. So on Wednesday the 15th of December, Dr. MH, PC, Smoking cessation- coordinator and PR, health link worker, along with the Mirpuri bilingual worker RR discussed the topic. Dr. MH took the lead on the discussion by explaining the religious, moral and social perspectives against smoking. He referred to the Quran and quoted Prophet Muhammad (PBUH) to highlight the advantages of giving up smoking. Although, there is no direct reference to smoking in the Quran, Islamic scholars have interpreted some verses in the Quran as instructing people about the social, economic and spiritual loss smoking brings.

However, at times, people have contested such interpretation and have advised Imams and health professionals to refrain from such acts. We had a listener who called into the show and asked for the proof for interpreting general verses of Quran in favour of very specific issues like smoking. Dr. MH, had a long justification for using Quranic verses this way.

In this connection, the following verses were mentioned to highlight the dangers and risks involved in smoking.

Do not kill (or destroy) yourselves for verily Allah (swt) has been most merciful to you|| *(4:29). And do not make your hands contribute to your destruction (2:195).*
Do not waste (resources) extravagantly (17:26).

While the health link worker dipped in and out of the discussion talking about the services available for giving up smoking, they left it to Dr. Hussian to do all the talking and allowed Islamic perspectives to take over the medical perspectives in the discussion. The health professionals were encouraged by the clear ideas of Dr. MH on the need for giving up smoking. They, in fact, asked him to refer members of his mosque to the Smoking Cessation team for guidance and advice. While this was a unique idea, how far people will talk to a religious leader whose views on smoking are very clear remains to be seen. However, a young lady rang in to explain her frustration with helping her CHD-patient father to give up smoking. She said she would do anything to support her father even take him to Dr. MH. She was told by the panel to seek a combination of heath advice, from both medical and spiritual points of view. There is evidence of this approach working in certain cases as is reported by Muslim Health Network, QUIT (British Heart Foundation's National Smoke Free Ramadan Campaign) and other smaller smoking cessation programmes undertaken in association with the local mosques in the UK. Similarly, the Muslim Council of Britain (MCB) and local primary care trusts have been working together for some time to help members of Muslim communities give up the habit of smoking.

The discussion on this particular show was more focused on how to support smokers to give up the habit, and social and cultural networks play a vital role in providing that help. Addictions and rehabilitation needs a multi-layered support which family, social networks, community organisations and health and wellbeing organization can provide, especially within the context of faith and culture.

Sexual Health and Sex Education

The first major publication in the UK about the Sex Education from Muslim points of view was authored by Mohammad Sarwar (1992). He argued that the 'majority of Muslim parents will be happy if there was no sex education at all in school' (1992:7). He found the education about contraception and abortion in conflict with the Islamic injunction which prohibits extra-marital sex. Sarwar goes further to question the secular and materialistic credentials of the British education system which he found to be ignorant about 'the spiritual and moral' aspects of life (1992: 11).

Many feel that sex education has become a lesson on the use of condoms which encourages promiscuity, resulting in abortions and sexually transmitted diseases. The government guidelines published in July 2000 warned of high rates of teenage pregnancy and sexually transmitted diseases and told schools that sex education should 'not encourage early sexual experimentation'. Similarly, a report from the

British Medical Journal (BMA, 2003) emphasized the need that schools must make greater efforts to address the growing incidence of sexually transmitted infections by including a more pro-active stance in warning about the risks of promiscuity and unprotected sex. Many Muslim adults find sex education in schools lacking moral and ethical perspectives, and Karimia Mosque was no exception.

We had an initial discussion on the topic, and SK was keen to open debate on sex education in the community. Through her network, she was able to find a Muslim doctor who specialized in Sexually Transmitted Diseases (STD). Dr. A was working as a specialist at the City Hospital in Nottingham and had strong views on people from minority ethnic groups trying to push everything under the carpet. Along with him, SN, a health outreach worker, joined Dr. MH in the discussion. However, it was difficult to convince Dr. MH to join the discussion because he felt uncomfortable with the concept of sex education, which he felt was carried out within a secular framework. While he was not averse to the need of talking about STD and other ailments linked with the human reproductive system, he was not keen to educate people on the sex. After long discussions with Dr. MH and Dr. A we decided that the topic itself will not be precisely about sex education but on sexual health, and if there were any inquiries from callers then Dr. MH will respond from the Islamic perspective while Dr. A will focus on the medical/clinical perspective.

This compromise was itself an achievement as a religious leader, a doctor and a health worker would take part in discussing the issues around sexual health/sex education. The show was as usual promoted for a few days before the actual broadcast. All the panellists on this show could speak either Mirpuri or Urdu and listeners were encouraged to ask questions to the panel. The show started with Dr. MH explaining the Islamic perspective on sex, children and family.

Highlighting the Islamic conceptualisation of sex life, he focused more on physical and physiological aspects and asked for a shift in understanding and education on sex and sexual health. He emphasized the need to have male teacher for boys and female teacher for girls to explain the anatomy of the human body. Dr. A first revealed the national and local figures about STD, followed by a medical explanation of various problems associated with sexual life. He encouraged parents to see health workers and their GP's to seek support and advice. He vehemently opposed the idea of pushing everything under the carpet:

> There is a stigma attached to the issues around sexual health but people from our community make things worse by not talking even to health professionals. There are many young men and women who are suffering in silence. They should not as there are confidential services available to people to help and support them. (Discussion on live Radio Show., Dec. 2000)

Health worker SN highlighted the role of health workers in signposting people to the appropriate places and persons and provided her details to encourage people to contact her. The show did not have as many callers as expected, but a few people left messages and asked questions off air. Most of the questions related to the fears and apprehensions parents had about the risks and dangers involved in sex education in mainstream schools to which both doctor and the health worker said that the parents have a choice, but Dr. A at the same time said that children are exposed to TV, films and Internet and they pick up things much earlier than their parents think`. He urged that if parents were not comfortable with sex education in schools they should start talking to them at home to help them avoid the risks and dangers. The debate got intense when a male caller rubbished the idea of preventing Muslim children from having sex education at a school. He argued that the number of 'unwanted pregnancies among the young Asians was on the increase and their parents were hiding their heads in the sand'.

Dr. MH asked the caller for evidence of this generalization and urged people to refrain from saying things which cannot be proved. This reaction from Dr. MH angered the caller who accused religious leaders of 'creating social problems by misleading innocent parents'. The debate went on for a while until Nilanjana intervened and asked the gentleman on the phone to contact her after the show. The caller was not satisfied and perhaps there were many more listeners like him.

While there is a case for teaching sex education in schools, but the questions many parents from the Muslim community are questioning the rationale behind such education. While the Western or mainstream point of view is to avoid underage sex, unwanted pregnancies and STD's, the fact is that the education on how to use a condom and what do after unprotected sex might encourage many young people to indulge in acts of promiscuity is something which worries many Muslim parents. This radio show at least opened an honest debate on the issue which many people do not want to hear. But we were surprised later to find out that the discussion on the topic was well received in the community. SN (health worker) was approached by many anxious parents to talk about the issues they could hardly talk to anyone else about.

Diabetes and Obesity

According to the National Service Framework for Diabetes, published in 2001, it is estimated that around 500,000 Diabetes sufferers in England are from Asian community. A large proportion of these Diabetic patients (six times more than white people) have Type 2 Diabetes, where cells are not able to produce enough insulin for the body's needs. It is also believed that Diabetes has a younger onset among Asians than whites, and is increasingly manifesting itself at young ages, including in children (Chaturvedi & Fuller, 1995).

It is believed that while some risk factors for developing Diabetes (such as family history, increasing age and ethnic origin) are non-modifiable, in many cases Type 2 Diabetes can be prevented, or its onset delayed, through sustained awareness and screening for early diagnosis. Besides having higher prevalence among people of South Asian origin, Diabetes is also found to be more common in socially deprived groups. This double disadvantage for people of South Asian origin creates complications, and with little awareness about the symptoms and implication of Type 2

Diabetes, these people become part of national statistics which suggest that the morbidity from Diabetes complications is three and a half times higher amongst the poorest people in England.

The programme on Diabetes had already generated some interest in the community because of the PSA which was broadcast in four languages (Mirpuri, Urdu, Bengali and English) five times a day. Before we went on air, people were sending their questions over the phone. So the show more or less became a question and answer session where people were asking specific questions about their conditions, and health professionals JP, SP and ST answered those questions. But the issues around lifestyle especially food and exercise, were coming in different ways into the show.

The approach of putting the blame on victims is seen by many as the offshoot of communitarian philosophy in which patients are made responsible for their behaviour and asked to perform and behave in a way that their lifestyle does not contribute to their ailments. There is a fund of literature available on the discourse of managerialism and medicalisation of health and well-being (for details see Chap. 5).

From the debates on Radio Ramzan it was evident that instead of being on a community radio, the debate on Diabetes was taking place within a familiar framework, and in order to break this circle, SK suggested the need to rethink the doctor-patient relation in which the patient is seen manifestation of illness and not a human being with a social and cultural context to his/her ailment. For example many South Asians, especially women, find it culturally inappropriate to go jogging in the public gaze, or to swimming in public baths and pools. Walking is one of the alternatives which some women of Mirpuri origin living in Forest Fields have found useful. The advice came from the show on Radio Ramzan which was followed up by the Mary Potter Health Centre. With the help of the Mirpuri health link workers, walking clubs were set up for the Asian community. The Forest recreation ground in Forest Fields has since become the hub for such walks which women take in groups to overcome inhibitions and fear of racial attacks due to their prominent dress.

Mental Health

Research suggests that people from minority ethnic groups living in the UK are more likely to be diagnosed with a mental health problem, admitted to hospital, experience poor outcome of treatment, and disengage from mainstream mental health service. The combination of these factors, along with experiences of racism, unemployment and poor housing, can lead to social exclusion which further deteriorates their mental health (Lloyd & Moodley, 1992; Goldberg, 1999). The statistics on the numbers of people of South Asian origin suffering from mental illness are inconsistent, though the prevalence of common mental health problems is seen as fairly similar across different ethnic groups, although rates are higher for Irish men and Pakistani women and lower for Bangladeshi women. While poverty, isolation and racism contribute to mental illness, it is believed that the mainstream mental health services often fail to understand or meet the needs of minority ethnic communities. These factors, when seen in combination with distrust of mental health services, mean that the people belonging to minority ethnic groups often seek professional help at a very late stage when their problems can be more serious. People from ethnic minority groups are six times more likely to be detained under the Mental Health Act than white people (Coid et al., 2000).

Health, according to the World Health Organisation's constitution, is 'a state of complete physical, mental and social well-being, not merely the absence of disease'. The report adds:

> *The health professions have largely followed a medical model, which seeks to treat patients by focusing on medicines and surgery, and gives less importance to beliefs and to faith – in healing, in the physician and in the doctor-patient relationship. This reductionism or mechanistic view of patients as being only a material body is no longer satisfactory. Patients and physicians have begun to realise the value of elements such as faith, hope and compassion in the healing process.*

Research also suggested that minority ethnic people, especially Muslims, find Western approaches to mental health treatment culturally inappropriate. While the majority of these people look for a holistic approach which takes into consideration the physical, emotional, mental and spiritual being, the mainstream services take a scientific approach. Scholars have for a while been arguing for working with the marginalised groups while the psychiatrists stress on conceptualisation of healing instead of cure to provide a holistic approach in dealing with mental illnesses.

Powell (2002) argues in favour of this theory in his paper 'Mental Health and Spirituality'. He says that the 'historical split between religion and science has had profound implications for the world we live in, culminating in a twentieth century culture modelled on the mechanistic, Newtonian paradigm of reality' (Powell, 2002: 1). He stresses that spiritual awareness should be the cornerstone of psychiatry along with the biological, social and psychological aspects of mental health. He argues that the spiritual dimension brings the prospect of healing (2002:10). In their important work on the issues of faith and mental health, Koenig, McCullough and Larson (2001) found that a sixty to eighty per cent correlation between religion or spirituality and better health was found in the areas of prevention, recovery and coping ability in a wide range of conditions. Faith and religious groups can offer a powerful opportunity to build positive social networks for people with mental health problems, and they can be particularly important for some ethnic minority groups. Research has shown that aspects of spirituality are linked with beneficial mental health outcomes and are consistently related to greater life satisfaction, happiness, morale and other indicators of well-being.

The social and cultural networks do offer a cushion that can help tide over the difficulties in life. The star presenter volunteer of Radio Ramzan, RS turned around his life from being an unemployed person to a Radio Jockey which ultimately helped him to find a job in the local partnership council. Here is his story in his own words:

I was not a brilliant student at school...dropped out and did odd jobs from selling double-glazing to mobile phone sim cards. Parents had expected me to do better. My father, a religious man, would send me to local mosque...but I did not find it stimulating there. I was confused...Radio has given me an opportunity to do something creative and at the same time serve my community and faith. When I got involved as a volunteer, I was a bit shy and could not take responsibility of presenting. I was more of a back stage support...would make tea and look after guests. With my experience from doing door to door selling, I started selling air time. I brought business for the radio station and got more and more involved. Then, I realized I could do a prog. We had Urdu background though my mother tongue is Poshtu. During one late night show, I did a bit of anchoring and liked it. There was immediate recognition which I could not get for years. Parents, friends and neighbours said it was fantastic. I had a boost to my confidence. I did more progs, and got involved in the management. I took a course at the Derby University in marketing. I was a new man. I developed contacts within the voluntary sector and became a member of the partnership council, started taking interest in wider community issues. Later a job for community outreach worker was advertised...I applied and got it. Rest is history. I am now on the management committee of the radio. (Excerpts from an Interview with RS, 2000)

It should be, however, recognized that every story cannot be like that of SR. While faith and spirituality can play a part, that is only a small part, as there are other social, financial and cultural issues which exclude many people. But for those who are isolated, elderly, and sick and who fear racial abuse, any support and comfort, from whatever source, can be helpful to overcome the agonies of mental illness. It is worth mentioning here that anecdotal evidence suggests that prevalence of higher social capital among Mirpuri/Pakistani communities is a myth and even in extended families people can feel lonely and neglected. The general attitude of health staff to exaggerate the family support in such cases reveals the lack of real insight, which is seen to be the main reason for the mainstream mental health services' failure to meet the needs of minorities' ethnic communities. As a health practitioner, SK had a good understanding of these issues, and through her network we involved Project Awaz- Asian mental health support group in Forest Fields, working with people of South Asian origin. Project Awaz has been advocating for appropriate mental health service for minority ethnic groups, using a community development approach and had established itself as the first point of contact for people suffering from mental illness, Project Awaz had already established links with various health agencies in the area and was in the forefront of raising awareness about mental health issues. ZF, chairman of the Awaz project was keen to develop his service further and to offer a comprehensive service for his clients in a comfortable environment in their mother tongues.

Although ZZF and his team were working for some time in Forest Fields, there was a lack of awareness among local people about the services and support offered by project Awaz. So in our first meeting I saw his enthusiasm to get involved in the HEAP project on Radio Ramzan.

Mental illness, being a highly stigmatized condition, is difficult to talk about, as many people who suffer from this disease are reluctant to come forward. Another difficulty was defining the mental illness and describing the conditions that can lead to mental health problems. After a few deliberations, it was decided to include conditions like stress, marital difficulties, failure, pressure, isolation/ loneliness, anxiety, and fear of racism in the causes of mental illness and developed a very broad framework for the debate. Issues like cultural sensitivity, access to services and language support were also included in this framework.

For the pertinent yet very sensitive issues of mental health issues among minority ethnic community, RR, Mirpuri bilingual worker and MSF, a local Imam were joined by Angela Kondola, a local mental health worker from the community group Awaz. The discussion opened the discussion by explaining the broader concept of mental health problems, specific symptoms and what services are available for those suffering from these problems. We had a phone call in the first ten minutes of the show. A lady living in Lenton rang and set the mood for the debate for the rest of the show. She was living with clinical depression for a long period of time and what prompted to ring her was to let everyone know how good she was feeling listening to Radio Ramzan. She gave graphic details of her loneliness and how radio was filling the void in her life. Speaking in Mirpuri language, she spoke of the problems of being a woman, an immigrant, a Mirpuri and having mental health problems. Her disadvantage was manifold. Much of what she was saying could fit into the life of a woman in any part of the world, but what made her situation worse was the fact that she had no support at home, could not speak English, and above all lacked the information on where to seek help.

When she was asked by ZH if she had heard of the project Awaz, the lady replied:

> *We do not hear of these projects and even if I did it would be difficult for me to reach where you are. My man would not allow me to go anywhere and he is bed-ridden. Your project is for those who can read and write. I am illiterate, cannot do anything. For me the big favour would be to have someone to talk to. I feel better talking to you in my own language…that's what I want.* (A caller on Radio Ramzan, Dec 2000)

The show continued and a few more callers were prompted to call in after listening to this lady. A caller commented that Mirpuri men would only let woman access mental health services if they are provided by local mosques as the groups are like Awaz were seen by some as 'corrupting woman'. This assertion was supported by the anecdotal evidence which suggested that Mirpuri men control every aspect of family life, even the choice of doctor and services that can be accessed. MSF emphasised the need to seek help from faith and spirituality under these circumstances and reminded listeners of the dangers of living in a 'soulless' Western society, which he described as being shallow and selfish. He said, 'Unless we bring purpose of helping each other and being just and God fearing, we will live isolated and greedy lives'.

In the beginning of this section we highlighted the role faith can have in helping people with mental health problems, and discussion on the radio again was revolving around cultural sensitivity, social appropriateness and acceptability. Reflecting on what was discussed on the show made me wonder if mosques and other community groups which are 'acceptable' to many within the community have the necessary capacity, resources and expertise to run such specialised services. More importantly, are these places welcoming to all, or just men who anyway are wielding a lot of power in a highly male-dominated society.

Public Service Announcement (PSA) on Health

As mentioned at the beginning of this chapter, one of the components of the HEAP project was the Public Service Announcement about the risks of CHD, Diabetes and Stroke among the South Asian population. The PSA was recorded in five languages and repeated five times a day to reinforce the message. This PSA was complementing the general discussions on these diseases and conditions.

The script of the PSA was written by a health professional but was vetted by the community and religious leaders to make it appropriate to local sensitivities, and at the end of this PSA telephone numbers of NHS Direct was given to help people contact this organisation for health needs. Although the service is believed to have been created to cut the queue time in hospitals and lessen the burden on GPs, in the case of HEAP the NHS Direct team acknowledged the health programme limitation and the inability to cover any given the subject matter in any depth other than raising awareness. However, after raising awareness, mechanisms needed to be in place which would enable more in-depth and individual support to be provided. This was made possible with the help and support of NHS Direct. This partnership was valuable both to HEAP and the NHS Direct. It provided an opportunity to NHS Direct, which is a fairly new service, to promote its service to the Asian community who are not aware of it. NHS Direct were involved in the early stages of the development of HEAP and the topics selected for the health programmes were discussed with them. This enabled the service to ensure resources and relevant translated material was available which could be posted out to people upon request. The service was promoted on a daily basis in English, Urdu, Bengali and Mirpuri and also during each health show. PSA Script:

> *Asians, especially Pakistanis and Bangladeshis have about 36 per cent higher chances of dying of Coronary Heart Diseases and 3 times higher chances of dying of Diabetes than the general population. Diabetes and high blood pressure increase the risk of heart disease and stroke. So it is important to visit a doctor or practice nurse if you develop symptoms such as thirst, passing more urine more frequently, unexplained weight loss or tiredness. High blood pressure does not usually give any symptoms. It can only be diagnosed when your blood pressure is measured. If you are over 35 years and have not had your blood pressure measured in the past three years, it is worth paying a visit to your doctor or practice nurse to have it measured. If you want to know more about Diabetes, heart condition, high blood pressure or any other illness, please ring NHS Direct on 0845 4647.*

Health Competition

Besides broadcasting live radio shows and playing health PSA, the HEAP Project also introduced a month long competition to facilitate public involvement in the project and develop stronger community partnership. Individuals and organisations were invited to produce a 10 minute recording of a health topic of their choice, relevant to ethnic minority communities. The following cash prizes were announced for this competition:

First Prize: 300 Second Prize: 200 Third Prize: 100 Runner up Prize: 50 (A flyer for promotion of this competition is enclosed as Appendix).Publicity for this competition began weeks before the start of Radio Ramzan through posters and flyers being distributed at local colleges, mosques, community centres and shops (Poster in appendix 3). The competition was also advertised on Radio Ramzan. A total of top five entries were shortlisted. Four entries were a monologue and one was a role play. One entry was in Urdu, one in Mirpuri and three in English on the following topics:

- Healthy Lifestyle Mirpuri 1st Prize
- Smoking cessation English 2nd Prize
- Travelling Abroad Urdu 2nd Prize
- Eczema English 3rd Prize Diet
- Exercise English Runner Up

The winning entries were played on Radio Ramzan, and the names of the winners of the competition were announced on the day of Eid (festival marking the end of fasting). The prizes were given out the winners at the HEAP seminar, which took place a week after the end of the Project and end of the transmission of Radio Ramzan.

Heap Seminar and Feedback Session

The last and crucial part of the HEAP project was the half day seminar, which was organized with the help of Karimia Mosque a week after the end of Ramadan. The main aims of the seminar were to:

- Provide service providers and users an opportunity for a face to face interaction
- Assess the impact of HEAP
- Collect listener feedback
- Identify gaps in service
- Propose a way forward

The announcements about this event were made while the radio station was still on air and in the last week of Radio Ramzan a big publicity campaign was run about this event. This radio publicity was supplemented with leaflets and posters which were distributed at the local mosques, community centres, taxi services, restaurant and take-aways in the city. The invitations to this seminar were extended to all Radio Ramzan listeners, contributors and guest speakers, key health policy leaders in the Health Authority and Local Authority, City Central PCT team and board members, local councillors and local community organisations.

Forest High School provided the appropriate venue for this seminar as it is centrally located and well known to the members of Mirpuri community living in Nottingham. On the day, various health and community organisations were invited to display to promote their services. Besides various health agencies, Nottinghamshire Police, Fire Services and the New Deal for Communities put up their stalls and information kiosks at the venue. The school wore a festive look as people flocked the venue. Over 150 attended the seminar including all Radio Ramzan volunteers, management committee members, and health professionals, members of other community organisations, local councilors and the representatives of businesses that supported the radio project.

Being a seminar on health education, the President of the Muslim Doctors and Dentists Association was invited to be the chief guest. His presence at the event added value and brought topicality to the whole project. In his speech he lauded the role of Radio Ramzan in bringing various health agencies and people together and making the month of Ramadan even more meaningful through a sustained health education campaign. He highlighted the role of Islam in developing the social, cultural, economic and wellbeing of the community, and urged mainstream health organisations to take full advantage of the faith-based organisations in reaching out to the minority ethnic groups to build their capacity to fight inequalities in health. The event also was unique in the sense that it offered fruits, salad and healthy snacks to the participants of the seminar which was a big contrast from the greasy and unhealthy food normally served on such occasions. After the food break, winners of the health competition were given their prizes and all the volunteers of Radio Ramzan were given certificates of merit for their involvement in the day to day running of the radio station.

Then came the big event of the day; the workshops to gain the audience feedback. For this purpose, four discussion groups were formed, led by a facilitator and supported with a scribe. There were two male and two female groups. All the discussions were bilingual or even trilingual using English/Urdu/Mirpuri. The turnout at the event was an indication that people liked the radio and had a sense of ownership of this community initiative. Over 150 people, mostly women, attended the seminar and took part in workshops. They were very vocal in their support for the station. Before we go into the details of the emerging themes from the focus group, here is a cross section of opinions, comments, and views of people collected at the seminar.

SK goes to the Claremont School in Sherwood and he thinks that Radio Ramzan has helped him to know more about himself:

> *We never used to listen to radio in our family...it was only TV and I was also watching cartoon shows...but Radio Ramzan has created a new past-time for me. To be honest, I did not know what is was all about...yes my parents would listen to it and we would open fast when they played Adhan, but for me to listen more attentively was when they started competition and they played some different music ... now it looks like Radio Ramzan is something we need...I know more about Mirpur where my grandparents have come from. I have been there only once when I was four...but now I want to go and know more about this place.*

A middle aged woman ZK put it this way.

> *'We felt we had a voice. The whole family would gather around radio, especially in the evenings. It made the month of Ramadan a real community thing'. Taking part in Radio Ramzan was seen as a proud moment, as people in both informal discussions and formally facilitated group discussions were reflecting on how everyone felt part of the community. The fact that the radio would relay the Adhan (call of prayers) at designated times, caught*

the attention of the whole community. The Adhan at dawn and dusk (start and completion of fast) was more important as it gave a sense of place and time to community. This central role of radio in creating a point of focus for the members of the Muslim communities in Nottingham is time and again mentioned at the seminar.

An 11 year-old student (SK) from New Basford said:

'My friends in Aspley and my cousin in Carlton would regularly listen to Bhajee Iffat's (Children's show presented by a popular teacher at the Forest Fields Primary School) show. Listening to the same show and calling in for competitions and reading poetry made me feel so proud. We would ring in one after another and our other friends from school would also join in. It was like one big family'. This sense of pride and being part of one big family is characteristic of small-scale localized media which people can easily relate to and feel part of. Being run in the month of Ramadan added more proximity to this station.

JK is a Math teacher and has been a regular listener of Radio Ramzan from the beginning:

It is a link, a sort of commonality...it has become a companion. It is about you and your own people ...bring Islam home. Radio has helped to gel people together at least for the listening pleasure...It has also helped me to listen to and look at other media more critically now. The discussions are best on this radio because we can hear a completely different point of view...the one which we do not normally hear on any other station. Though, about this point of views in private, radio has brought these debates into the public.

Radio *Ramzan* did not come into existence all of a sudden. There is a whole context against which this radio station evolved. The exclusion and disadvantage faced by the members of Mirpuri community, and being left out in the mainstream media discourse rendered these communities disillusioned at the peripheries. The need for cultural and social support to overcome exclusion led the members of this community to look inwards for support. While mosques and other community institutions were offering a space to engage with communal and local issues, the radio station was seen a community-wide platform to raise awareness and generate debates to support faith-based initiatives to fight exclusion. Many alternative media movements draw inspiration from the Gramscian concept of counter-hegemony to 'generate alternatives in public debate' and to oppose the 'agency of domination'. The 'common sense' and 'taken for granted' view of hegemony, which legitimizes the interest of the bourgeoisie as 'natural' is disrupted and questioned by the very presence of alternative points of view (Downing, 2001: 15-16). Although identity formation is a contested concept, it is very much associated with peoples' rituals, cultural practices and traditions. Werbner (2005:19) sees this association as a 'mode of the transaction and relatedness', as well as a 'discursive imaginary of selfhood, identity, subjectivity and moral virtue'. Whether identity formation is the capacity to draw attention to the issues of 'representation' (Hall, 1997), or the tendency to gravitate towards a 'shared culture' (Desai, 1963) or an expression of 'socio-cultural particularism' (Raghuram, 1999), it needs tangible spaces and contexts where people can express their group and collective aspirations. For members of Muslim communities, while mosque provides a spiritual and social space, the festivals like Ramadan (month of fasting) provide the context for Muslims to formulate, practice and express their way of life.

MI, a local councilor and former Lord Mayor of Nottingham, captured the essence of how this radio station provided a common frame of reference despite the difference within the community:

We have differences, and that is the way things are. We would hardly engage in debates to explore these differences to find some ground for collective action on issues that affected us all. Take the example of Muslim burial ground or state funded Islamic school in Nottingham. We remain divided...We still have differences of opinion but at least we're talking now. With Radio Ramzan on air, people with different affiliations and loyalties were voicing their concerns which otherwise was not possible. With nearly a dozen mosques and an even higher number of community and political groups operational in the city, it was always difficult to bring people together to talk. Consequently, everyone was working within their own circles...I have many differences with the way Karimia Mosque is run, but the radio station created a space beyond the walls of mosques and community groups, and for the time, I felt we were talking on a common ground. (MI, 2000)

Note

1. The Community Radio Association (CMA) is the umbrella organisation of many broadcasters, activists, academicians, social workers and community workers joining hands to mobilize public opinion in favour of decentralisation of broadcasting through establishment of community based radio stations that increase participation and involvement at local level. The Community Media Association (CMA), formerly known as the community radio association was founded in 1983. The CMA is a membership organisation open to individuals and organisation.

Chapter 7
Agency, Identity and Empowerment

This study, as a pedagogy of inclusion, explored the multiple connections between agency, identity and social mobility. In doing so, the project took a contextual approach, and looked at the issues of marginalisation from the intersection of various disciplines and perspectives which helped to take this research closer to peoples' day to day lives and their cultural practices. Working on the premise that in many post-industrial Western cities, a complex relationship between social conditions, geographic location and the ethnic and racial background of people create a culture of disadvantage, this developed a multi- disciplinary framework that allowed the people's experiences, knowledge and points of views to develop a dynamic and engaging theory which opened up the ways for thinking outside the disciplinary rigidities and essentialist reading of community and communication. This framework, on the one hand, helped to raise a critical consciousness about the causes and consequences of marginalisation, and on the other explored the possibilities of dealing with it.

The case study of the Health Education Awareness Project (HEAP) campaign on Radio Ramzan, which brought into focus the inequalities in health faced by the people belonging to the Mirpuri community living in inner city Nottingham, helped to ground the concept of communication as a process of social interaction for sharing experiences and formulating actions. Although this was not a straight- forward process, as many conflicts came to the surface, the radio station, however, provided the context for the members of the Mirpuri community to engage through mediated and interpersonal communication to reproduce and represent their shared interest. It will be naïve to assume though, that the community-based communication initiatives like Radio Ramzan can offer solutions to the complex problems of social exclusion but, as was demonstrated during the month of Ramadan, the radio station provided a context for sharing and legitimizing experiences at a wider platform. Radio Ramzan, as a communitywide platform, assisted in the formation, maintenance and propagation of solidarities and identities among people who share interests in terms of faith, country of origin and kinship. It was not only a platform that

F. Malik, *Addressing Health Inequalities through Community Media*,
https://doi.org/10.1007/978-3-031-35237-9_7

debated the bigger issue but it also helped people to keep a focus on the everyday life matters like sharing information on cultural events, car boot sales, births, deaths, funerals, weddings, lost and found, and so on. This was possible in a situation where the medium was embedded in the social and cultural life of the community it served.

A number of similar studies across the world have demonstrated that participatory media encourage 'cultural humanity' that have the potential to become a viable cultural resource to facilitate positive interventions and support developmental capacities for public campaigns addressing specific issues within a group or community (McLeroy et al., 2003; Huppert, 2009; Knibbe et al., 2017). The small scale media, like community and other forms of alternative media, are thought to be a vital counterbalance to a media landscape which is seen as 'Habermasin refeudalisation of the public sphere' in which legislations and business models stifle alternative voices (Saeed, 2009). While at the global level the powerful transnational media networks, using financial muscle and new technologies, create global audiences, at a very local level, people who feel the need to raise and discuss their very local issues, find use local networks and cultural practices to debate and disseminate information relevant to them. There are numerous examples of the phenomenon where people develop their own media rather the people being made into passive audiences. In the developing world, there is a strong tradition of folk media, which along with puppetry, theatre, poetry and religious songs have been used over centuries for communicative interaction within small groups. The study of media with community rather than communication as the focus is taking place against the background of the `theoretical shift from a persuasion model to one based on cultural democracy, from a transmission to an empowerment process, and from a linear to a two-dimensional model (Dagron, 2001; McQuail, 1994). Putting forward the democratic theory of communication, McQuail explains that the shift in our understanding of the communication process is taking place when new communication technologies are challenging the standardized, commercialised and professionalised mass media. In the wake of these developments, he envisages small-scale local, non-profit making, media engages sender and receiver into a meaningful process where the horizontal pattern of communication is preferred over a linear model. McQuail placed the media in both the developed and developing world under this criticism to favour small-scale media for facilitating horizontal patterns of interaction (McQuail, 1994: 132). In retrospect, the debates over the role of communication in development has moved from understanding communication as a 'linear information transmission/diffusion process' to support modernisation (Shannon & Weaver, 1949; Lerner, 1958; Schramm, 1964) to conceptualising communication as a process of 'shared meaning' that is inseparable from the context; a process of resistance, empowerment and freedom (Boderave & Diaz, 1977; Zimmerman & Rapport, 1988; Crush 1995). The dialogic process as is thought to be key to such emancipatory communication, which 'enables participants to identify and explore issues that a common meaning for them' (Melkote & Steeve, 2001: 39). These media entail a radical change in the creation, production, distribution and the whole process of the communication practice with a focus on empowerment and action (Couldry, 1999; Atton, 2001; Atton & Couldry, 2002).

Scholars influenced by political economy have developed a comprehensive and consistent critique of the commercial use of media, which they believe reduces choice and concentrates power into fewer hands. In the famous book Manufacturing Consent Edward Herman and Noam Chomsky take a detailed look at the propaganda model of mass media, arguing that the rich and powerful, including governments and special interest groups, influence the news agenda through ownership, advertising, public relations, disciplining and anti-communism (1988:2). Within this approach, it is argued that the lines between producers and users of information blur as audiences take a more proactive role, creating a mutual relationship between alternative media and the social movements (Downing, 2003). This also gives disenfranchised and marginalized communities 'presence' and 'agency' to democratize the media (Downing, 2001:5–6). The group dialogue is seen by many critical scholars as crucial in communication strategies for liberation to advance empowerment and solidarity. Atton and Couldry (2002) sees these practices working alongside the reflexive practices that emerge from owning, establishing and producing alternative visions of participation, power and action.

As was observed during the Health Education awareness Project on Radio Ramzan, the initiative facilitated non-mediated communication among and across the members of the community as the discussions and debates on this radio carried on in streets, Malls, social gatherings and cultural events. This cascading effect of community-based medium reached far due its cultural and social proximity which was enhanced by the topics of discussion, languages and dialects used, familiarity of radio presenters and above all participation of local businesses and voluntary groups to support this station. Many a times taxi drivers, restaurant owners, local grocers would be seen heard getting involved in debates post program broadcasts. In the local shopping centre in Forest Fields, elderly men and women from the community were seen discussing and giving their own opinions on health issues debated on radio night before. While the author was in a queue at the grocery shop, there was an animated discussion between a group of women on what is the best food for people suffering from diabetes. This discussion was initiated by the radio program they heard their own language (Mirpuri dialect of Punjabi) with a local general practitioner and health education specialist. The author was on many occasions asked by the taxi drivers to elaborate on the topics while on a ride in Nottingham and further requested for questions to be asked on their behalf to different experts. Such experiences while being very heartening to the author indicated how a locally owned and operated platform can generate a participation seldom seen in mainstream media. This way community media provided a common ground, within a familiar social setting, for the interaction between mediated and interpersonal communication to serve as a frame of reference for a shared interpretation of the relevance of the topics communicated within the community (Hollander & Stappers, 1992: 19–20)

Many alternative media movements draw inspiration from the Gramscian concept of counter-hegemony to 'generate alternatives in public debate' and to oppose the 'agency of domination'. The 'common sense' and 'taken for granted' view of hegemony, which legitimizes the interest of the bourgeoisie as 'natural' is disrupted and questioned by the very presence of alternative points of view (Downing, 2001: 15–16) The defiance to the dominant through counter-hegemony is analysed by Downing in his seminal work on new social movements and alternative media. He stresses the 'dialectical' relationship and 'interdependence' of New Social Movements (NSM) and radical media, arguing that both 'represent dynamic expressions of resistance' (Ibid: 23–24). This is not to suggest that the grassroots/community radio mode is not without its inconsistencies and contradictions. It is believed that alternative use of media could easily be subverted and co-opted from its democratic origins to become another monopoly of knowledge. In embracing local cultures and indigenous knowledge systems, there is a danger that community radio can perpetuate hidden forms of violence such as the continued exploitation of women or destruction of the natural environment in the guise of being inherently good because it is an alternative to the dominant model. There is a danger that in the struggle to create new forms of participatory communications, the same pattern of inequalities and injustices of the dominant model are replicated. Downing (2001:34) warns that an uncritical populist way of referring to community as a 'seamless social tissue that is local and, therefore, healthy' could lead to making 'idiotic assumptions about the absence of class and other serious rifts within the local tissue'. Accepting the fuzziness that shrouds the concept, Downing (2001), however, cannot think of any alternatives that can represent all that the concept encompasses:

> *It is, therefore, exceptionally hard to give the term community a lucid and exact sense. Yet when the word is used as convenient verbal shorthand for the spectrum of the relatively dispossessed or local realities, it is hard to think of a replacement.* (Ibid: 39)

Whatever shape debate on the concept of the community takes, one cannot escape the fact that media at the local /communal level are seen as institutions expressing demands and priorities from below, from those excluded and those who are powerless. Inherent to these arguments is the idealistic notion of such media as egalitarian or democratic. However, they can create the local replica of corporate power and serve as instruments of the very hegemonic structures and processes they are seen as opposed to, or give more voice to already vocal local elite, which can further stifle the voiceless. Downing (2001: 40), warns that such media 'may easily conceal more than they reveal'. However, one cannot deny the power of such media in helping local communities in fostering and facilitating dialogue and building their capacity to fight the institutions and processes that dis-empower and exclude them. Local and community based media are an effective means in acting as loudspeakers, but there are more important and effective webs of interpersonal communication networks that have a role in and outside the public sphere. Downing (2001) recognizes the role of such networks as essential both to such media and to the social and political movements. Acknowledging that these networks can operate independently of the media, he argues that such networks can be fed by, or can feed into, alternative media. Within the context of social movements, public sphere, communication networks and alternative media, he argues that the usefulness of communication networks is that they help to 'get away from the notion of audiences as atomized, composed simply of individuals or households and underscores the internal connectivity of social movements'. He further argues that within this conceptualization the public sphere is more than an idealized platform but more a space for mutual communication at various levels and points.

The emancipatory use of media is believed to help in 'collective mobilization' through a decentralized and interactive process (Enzensberger, 1974) with emphasis on 'communication rather than on distribution system' (Brecht, 1983: 169). Within this framework, community based media are seen to harness the 'cultural identity' of local people, and facilitate their 'participation' (Servaes, 1999: 88). Many scholars, mostly coming from critical perspectives, have underlined the importance of small-scale media that help facilitate an informed debate. Historically, these media have evolved from the critique of the state and the corporate uses of communication (Wasko & Mosco, 1992). Although the debate on the role of communication in development has for long stressed the need for context, access and participation, the use of Western models and over-reliance on technology is thought to have taken focus away from the structural, institutional and cultural determinants that breed and reinforce inequality and exclusion (Escobar, 1995a, b; Melkote & Steeves, 2001). The exclusion and disadvantage faced by the members of Mirpuri community, and being left out by the mainstream media (see Chaps. 2 and 4) had long left this community disillusioned. The need for cultural and social support to overcome exclusion led the members of this community to look inwards for support. While mosques and other community institutions were offering a space to engage with communal and local issues, the radio station was seen a community-wide platform to raise awareness and generate debates to support faith-based initiatives to fight exclusion.

The discursive aspect of power relations help to understand how an individual may be positioned or subjectified in restrictive ways by others. The positioning by the mainstream media of those who live on the margins can be understood by analyzing the process through post-structuralism. But this process should not be seen as irreversible as within the paradigm of alternative media, this subjectification moves to a more privileged position where being on the margin is not abnormal or a deviation but another way of being. Within post-structuralism, identity or subjectivity is understood to transpire through one's positioning. This gives the individual a privilege as an active agent rather than passive object (Lowe, 1998: 207). Looking at the example of Radio Ramzan, it was found that people get involved for various reasons: loyalty, compassion, conviction and so on. Emotions and feelings play a big part in such participation. The emotions, which gear individual and collective involvement, are subjective, chaotic and weak but are believed to ignite creative energy and involvement (Putnam & Mumby, 1993:4). Whether one feels discriminated against or marginalized, the feelings of being not treated fairly makes people think of alterative institutions and means to resolve issues. The 'expanded consciousness' (Freire, 1972) that initiates action has been argued to be critical to 'democratic participation and empowerment' (Zimmerman & Rappaport, 1988), endorses validation of peoples' knowledge and influence on the issues that affect them as fundamental in increasing participation. This way communicative interaction becomes a part of the process of democratization (Melkote & Steeves, 2001).

Ownership of the process to make choices based on one's experiential knowledge underlines both agency and structural approach to address inequalities (Kabeer, 1999). This empower-centred approach is also present in a number of policies and declaration (WHO, 1986, 1997). The lack of such influence is seen a 'risk factor' while having ownership and health initiative is mostly conceived a strategy that can improve health (Wallerstein, 1992)

The Health Education Awareness Project on Radio Ramzan, which chronicled a month-long health education campaign, engaged social aspects of life with the spiritual to develop a unique health promotion programme in which members of the local Muslim communities entered into debates and discussions about situation to develop initiatives for empowerment through critical reflection and collective action. The project focused on the most pertinent health problems within this community which include Coronary heart diseases, Diabetes and Obesity, Mental Health, Smoking, and sexual health in a unique partnership with public and voluntary sector to mobilize community and increase their participation in the campaign. The process of conceiving and delivering the HEAP project involved developing strategies to bridge the gulf between theory and practice. While the project had broad goals of participation and empowerment set as guiding principles, it was the actual practice of situating these principles within the faith, culture and experiences of marginalized people that made the process meaningful, and it was this power of contextual participatory communication that enabled the journey towards achieving social, cultural and gender empowerment. The radio station in general and the health awareness project, run on this station, in particular developed the capacity of the local people to express their concerns, develop a boarder consensus and run a campaign their rights. Though health and wellbeing remained the focus of the campaign, the project demonstrated that health can not to be taken in isolation from other social, economic and cultural realities people live in.

The radio project in Nottingham substantiated these arguments as people's involvement in a dialogic process, which started well before the actual broadcasting and did not end even after the radio was off the air. Within the participative paradigm, community-based media enable the involvement of people in the conception, production and the evaluation of the content, thereby offering ways and means for the voices to be heard. There by a social context was created to the spiritual life, and through this equation of social with the spiritual, the station promoted a holistic approach to community development where people's references to their culture and faith complemented their efforts to fight social exclusion. This was best demonstrated by the month-long health education campaign, Health Education Awareness Project (HEAP) on Radio Ramzan wherein the religious leaders, health professionals and the community workers shared a common platform to raise health awareness within a religious and culturally sensitive context. This approach provided the legitimacy to health education as radio facilitated the individual and the community participation via a sustained interaction. The HEAP campaign demonstrated the fact that a health education programme can have a long-term dividend and enjoy wide support from people if it acknowledges and adapts to the cultural practices of people and respects their points of view. Keeping in view the marginalization, cultural and social impediments, service health service users from minority ethnic groups face, this experience was unique as the premises of a faith based organization, and a platform owned by local people brought service providers to the service users, and let them discuss and find ways of addressing the issues of approach and access within a familiar environment for the users. FR, a community worker from Forest field and member of Radio Ramzan team, captured this aspect of radio:

> *All the issues raised on Radio Ramzan whether social, political or economic are interrelated and have an impact on health. So you cannot put health in that medical box...it is all connected. Radio Ramzan helped to look at health as a whole and not just from the clinical point of view. This is important for a community that is disadvantaged and faces inequalities in health. I remember some of the issues touched in the HEAP programmes were picked up by other programmes and there was continuing debate on the following day. In fact the debates were not confined to radio only. As a community worker I know how these discussions cascaded down. The month of Ramadan added values to these debates. The shows on sex education, mental health and smoking had a better reception as the Karimia Mosque gave the health education campaign the much need cultural legitimacy and social proximity.*

The study reinforced the fact that health and well-being cannot be divorced from other elements of human development as it affects every other capability. It was found that much of the work into inequalities in health has paid little attention to the social, cultural and political aspects of life by over-simplifying the very complex nature of community, ethnicity and identity, and through the racialisation of health of minority ethnic groups. Against this background, the insights from intersectionality, power relations and critical consciousness helped to map the contours of health inequalities from the victims point of view and looked at how the racial background of many minority ethnic groups has become 'etiologically important in the development of illness' (McKenzie, 2003; Karlsen & Nazroo, 2002).

A counter argument to this 'pathologising' of race, ethnicity and difference, the study learning from the various forms of cultural expression of marginalized groups, offered valid sites of analysis to shift the focus from a clinical view of health to a more holistic approach in dealing with inequalities in health. This provided the basis for the evaluation of the HEAP project as a campaign grounded in the subjective experiences of people, especially their relationship with their spirituality. By theorizing this dynamic link between the social and spiritual, the study conceived an empowering and sustainable way in foregrounding people in the fight against the inequalities. The theorization proved critical in moving away from the state 'managed' conceptualisation of health to a holistic approach based on people's participation and knowledge.

There is no doubt that the HEAP campaign had many lessons for the community as well as for the local NHS Trust but, as happens with most of the community-based partnership projects, there was no sustainability. While it looked good on paper for the Health Department to show off their commitment in fighting health inequalities, in reality it raised expectations of people, and those expectation were not met. As the feedback session revealed, people said it was a good project but 'what now'? It will be unfair not to mention the inherent deficiencies within the voluntary/community sector, which lacks the capacity and organizational structure to take on such projects on a long-term basis. The local politics, power struggles and more importantly the competition for limited resources proved major bottleneck for sustaining the projects. But one cannot deny the fact that it helped to conceive and develop a unique approach to health promotion. The study exhibited the need to reflect not only on how to overcome the barriers at the service user's end but, more importantly, at the service provider's end, whose own attitudes, assumptions, notions and practices could be contributing to perpetuating rather than eliminating health inequalities.

As was effectively exhibited during the month of Ramadan, Radio Ramzan, situated within the religious ethos, enhanced the reach and access of the health campaign. This, however, should not mean that the use of cultural practices, especially faith, should be appropriated to make the process of fighting inequalities and exclusion attractive. In this study the sole idea of having people in the driver's seat is to help people develop strategies to deal with their own social realities through human agency and dialogical praxis. Radio Ramzan, despite its short-term nature, demonstrated that it can facilitate participation, especially among the marginalized communities, reducing the risks of isolation and exclusion. The radio station proved to have the potential of a sustainable voice for the silenced groups to speak up in their own languages, build confidence, develop actions and play a decisive role in their own empowerment.

This process is important for the people who are not only marginalised by the mainstream media, but often demonized through a media discourse that particularly is disrespectful to Muslim life and their cultural practices. This projection of incorrect images based on pre-conceived notions, racism and prejudice has come to be known together as Islamophobia (Fredman et al., 2001). In 1997, the Runnymede Trust defined Islamophobia as the 'dread or hatred of Islam and therefore, to the fear and dislike of all Muslims,' stating that it also refers to the practice of discriminating against Muslims by excluding them from the economic, social, and public life of the nation.

This study has deliberately omitted the discussions on 9/11 and 7/7 as these events fall outside of the period remit (July 1997–July 2001) of the thesis. However, it is worth mentioning here that, not surprisingly, these events have both impacted significantly upon a number of the issues raised throughout, particularly the issues of exclusion because of the negative perception of Muslims in the media and general public and the self-image of Muslims in the community. This case study of Radio Ramzan, however, will serve as a precursor to what was happening within the Muslim communities in the UK before 9/11. This study hopes to serve as a reference for the comparisons in Muslim/minority politics before and after 9/11 as it records in detail the growing significance of thesmosque in the social life of Muslim communities and an emerging aspiration to assert their 'own' worldview. Although it will be naïve to link these aspirations to what has been labelled as the 'radicalization of Muslim youth' in the UK, the disillusionment with mainstream institutions, especially the media, was evident from this study. Radio Ramzan, though a temporary initiative, provided hope to the people that 'owning and running our own media' is possible.

As an action research project, the study put the theory about the efficacy of small scale and communally-focused community media into practice, and in the process learnt about the possibility of employing the narrative of dialogic communication for raising consciousness and developing agency. The month-long project demonstrated that informed discussions grounded in people's knowledge and experience can improve the ability of the members of the community to raise problems, analyze them, and work together to solve them. This blended approach became not just a process of sharing knowledge but also generating knowledge as the receivers of the information were actively engaged in the production of content for this radio station. The exclusion and disadvantage faced by the members of the Mirpuri community along with the disengagement from the mainstream institutions, especially the mainstream media, has left this community disillusioned. The need for cultural and social support to overcome these disillusionments has led the members of this community to look inwards for support. While various community institutions, including the mosques and charities do help people to engage locally and communally, the radio station offered a community-wide tool to reach out to members of the community to work together. This generated a sense of camaraderie and people, organizations and local businesses came forward to provide social, institutional and financial resources needed to sustain this project. The resources, like time and skills from dozens of volunteers, proved valuable social capital, while the resources including the space for studio, telephone, computers and furniture from the local mosque and book shop came as vital institutional support. Similarly, the financial support through donations, sponsorships and advertising from local taxis, take-aways, books shops, boutiques and jewelers kept the daily operations going. These resources not only made the broadcasting possible for 30 days round the clock but also enhanced the communitarian feeling.

When a listener from the West Bridgford area of Nottingham volunteered to do the sound- proofing of the studio after many people complained about the bad sound quality, more people came forward and offered both material and in-kind support to make this community project a success. Similarly, one morning on the breakfast show, our usual receptionist did not turn up, and the presenter appealed on air for support to take phone calls. Within fifteen minutes of this appeal three people living in the vicinity of the studio on Radford Road turned up at the station to look after the reception. This proximity is difficult to observe both in public service and commercial broadcasting anywhere. People spoke in their mother tongues without the fear of being excluded, and they enjoyed learning basics of production and presentation though peer education. This learning was very informal and pedagogic in which the teachers and learners shared the same passion and operated within the same discursive space. Ordinary people's voices could be heard, debating issues and posing questions to those who exercise authority. The Imam of the local mosque, the local councillor and the doctor from the local surgery were sharing airwaves with the members of Mirpuri community. The language and the localness of the issues discussed, enhanced the proximity as the debates on radio were heard cascading down to shops, schools and social and communal gatherings. Being a presenter myself, the author was approached many times and was given spontaneous feedback.

Radio Ramzan provided a voice, both in reality and symbolically to help people to propagate and validate their own knowledge and worldviews. The communicative interaction facilitated by this radio station in practice is described by critical scholars as 'participation through media' for self-representation in the public spheres for collective decision making (Couldry, 2003). The intersectionality, as promoted within the feminist scholarship, provided an analysis to conceptualise the interrelatedness and multiplicity of forms of disadvantages and discriminations. The very presence of RR, the health practitioner on Radio Ramzan, encouraged many other women to join discussions. RR was not only a health worker but was also a practising Muslim, a Mirpuri woman who was born and brought up in the Forest Fields area of Nottingham. Her passion about the issues of patriarchy within the Mirpuri community, the voicelessness and racialised identity of Muslim women on the one hand, and her determination to change the practice of health education on the other, had a positive effect on the HEAP campaign. She understood local women's issues as well as the problems and prejudices of the practice of health promotion. This epistemological privilege helped the study to challenge the positional superiority of Western knowledge for its failure to engage with the life and experience of 'other' women. At the same time, this position offered a unique analysis by bringing Mirpuri womens interpretation of identities, experiences and power relations to the centre of the debate on health inequalities. RR's presence helped to ground theory of feminism contextually in the day to day lives of marginalized people (Stacey, 1988). It would be, however, wrong to suggest that the radio station had solutions to all the issues and problems faced by the members of excluded communities in Nottingham. Radio Ramzan was a time-bound experiment which exhibited its potential in generating alternative voices but, at the same time, revealed a number of deficiencies in this project including the gendered nature of the station, the dominance of religious elite and the divisions and difference of opinions within the community itself. Some voices of dissent could be heard from the fringes of the community as not everyone was in favour of having this radio station run from the local mosque.

But in the absence of a radio station these feelings and contestations would have remained out of the public debate. The community-based project, specifically, cannot claim to have the complete involvement of all people or give representation to all shades of opinion all the time. To make such a claim will be misleading. Radio Ramzan, as has been stated in the introduction to this thesis, emerged against the backdrop of a number of conflicting realities and multiplicities on the one hand, and the common experiences of marginalisation and discrimination on the other. The radio station, in fact, reconciled through some of these multiplicities using the process of dialogic communication. The study demonstrated the explicit subjectivity and intention of offering a situated version to the various possibilities of knowledge and knowing. One such possibility came through Radio Ramzan when it gave expression to many voices and opinions which normally remain stifled and bottled-up due to lack of alternative platforms and forums. But the dissent and difference of opinion is not only due to the affiliations to various schools of thought or links with particular groups, clans and political organizations. The Muslim communities are largely seen to be patriarchal where rights of women are violated in the name of tradition and validated in the name of culture (Afkhami, 1999). While it is debatable whether patriarchy is intrinsic to Islam or is part of Muslim cultures and geographies (Ahmad, 2003), the gendered nature of Muslim organizations which are dominated by men is widely accepted.

While it was beyond the scope of this thesis to engage into the debates about Islam and gender issues, however, the gendered nature of Radio Ramzan, which claimed to be the voice of the Mirpuri community in Nottingham, came under scrutiny in different ways. Although, around 25 per cent of the presenters on the Radio Ramzan were women and there was also an exclusive show, 'Sisters Hour' for them during day time, all the discussions and debates were taking place within a patriarchal framework. In the majority of the shows, these women were discussing their roles as mothers, wives, daughters and sisters, and there was little about the issues they face as women in the gendered society they lived in. However, for the first time in their lives, women had a chance to raise and discuss issues. This was a big change from a position where women have to listen and follow. The women of Mirpuri origin are not just the victims of patriarchy but the fact that they are non-white, immigrant and belonging to socially excluded groups, adds to their disadvantage.

Besides the socio-economic empowerment, there was a marked shift towards women empowerment where the women from the community would campaign for their 'voice to be heard within and outside the community. There were a number of women working as researchers, presenters and producers on the station but there was always that uneasiness in working in a male dominated studio and management structure. The discussion was not about equality but more of a proactive approach in having an agency within the community to express, find solidarities and eventually create gender sensitive solutions. Without giving this undercurrent a label of feminism, these women did not want activism but within their culture wanted their own frameworks and systems. The voice of a separate women radio station started getting stronger even during the broadcast and the 'Sisters Hour' show was becoming more of a platform to bring out the issues from domestic violence to sexism to racial discrimination and male domination.

This all was happening when women in general and those of immigrant South Asian origin were facing an essentialised discourse in media, academia and public policy. They are objectified and stereotyped which trivializes their existence. In many ways, this perception leads to 'othering' of women of colour who face disadvantage as being part of the immigrant, inner city, unemployed, and having poor health. So, facing a double disadvantage, women of south Asian origin had an opportunity to challenge their situated existence in mainstream discourse while championing for their own framework within a highly patriarchal community. Eventually, these women organized under the banner of Asian Women's project and applied for a license to run their own radio station in Nottingham. This led to the establishment of Radio Kiran, the first women radio station in the UK. The station operated from Forest Fields area of Nottingham for women to organize and express themselves, and provided volunteering opportunities for women in a familiar setting to develop their skills in a culturally appropriate environment. The radio station started broadcasting in August 2000 within a secular ethos in contrast to Radio Ramzan which operated within a religious framework. After the completion of the restricted broadcast for a month, the Asian Women's team applied for

This implies that participation becomes meaningful and empowering when there is a shift from the media to the people and from persuasion to participation. This paradigm shift cannot take place within the existing mass media where the whole emphasis, in the war of ratings, is on increasing numbers; on quantity rather than on quality. While the BBC is not commercial in the sense that it does not allow advertising on its domestic services, it follows the principles of commercial media to determine its popularity. It uses the Radio Joint Audience Research (RAJAR) figures to show how many people are listening to its services. While the commercial stations use these figures to determine their advertising rates, the BBC uses them to justify license fees which every British resident pays. Many people 'othered' due to their immigration status, cultural background, ethnicity, sexual orientation and socio-economic ability, are further pushed to the margins in this ratings war by both the commercial and the public service media.

In the beginning many women groups including the Asian Women Project (AWP) and Muslim Women Organisation (MWO) along with Muslim women professionals like teachers, health workers and social workers from Nottingham were invited in the open meetings to give women representation in the management and running of this month-long radio station. But only one woman was actually on the management committee. The AWP and MWO did take part in programme production and presented regularly on Radio Ramzan but there were many tensions between these two groups of women. While Radio Ramzan had assumed the role of being the sole representative of the Muslim community in Nottingham, some women volunteers of the station challenged that claim by setting up Radio Kiran (Ray of light) to represent the 'voice of Asian Women' under the banner of Asian Women's Project (AWAP). Radio Kiran started broadcasting in August 2000 and opened up the possibility of other points of view which were over-shadowed by the male dominated Radio Ramzan. In fact, Radio Kiran went further to promote this radio station as a voice for Asian women to include non-Muslim women of South Asian origin including Hindus and Sikhs and people of Gujarati and Bangladeshi origin. The fact that a womens group managed to get the license, develop the resources and operated a radio station in the territory of the dominant Muslim radio station, demonstrates the relational and discursive nature of power which is not always repressive. Although, Radio Ramzan obscured the gendered nature of the Mirpuri community, the fact that this radio station was the first Muslim organization to recognize the need to involve women, gave them some hope and encouragement. It was due to the exposure on Radio Ramzan (though limited), that women started their own station.

From the gender point of view, another interesting feature of Radio Ramzan was that the majority of its listeners were women. The evidence gathered from the phone calls received and the head count at the final feedback session revealed that women made up a substantial part of the audience of Radio Ramzan. It was found that for the illiterate, isolated and voiceless women (mostly confined to the four walls of their houses), the radio station became a purposeful companion. It was for the first the time that women of Mirpuri origin were articulating issues on a community-wide platform. Having a limited say in the public affairs, this was the first time womens voices could be heard in the public space and many women found it empowering. In this regard the HEAP project played a significant role. The discussions in the Mirpuri language, the presence of a Mirpuri health professional (RR) along with the familiar context of Karimia Mosque helped women to identify with what was being said. RR was already known to many of these women. Her inside-knowledge proved an asset to the success of this campaign. She co-produced and co-presented the shows, and played a critical part in the self-reflections after every show. My association with her helped me to understand the issues from a very unique perspective.

Problematising the concept community has been an important part of this study. This meant to critically examine the seamless and egalitarian notions of community on the one hand, and on the other to look at the dynamic process of formation and fragmentation of the community. The critique of the notion of community benefited from the poststructuralist analysis of subjectivities and power relations. Poststructuralism, especially Foucauldian analysis recognizes the construct of community as a series of discursive relationships engaging with shifting perspectives of race, ethnicity, religion, politics and immigration. During the research process, the power tussles, silencing, and labelling were reflected through the discourses of patriarchy, essentialism and racism within the disadvantaged Mirpuri community. Foucauldian analysis was helpful in finding centres and peripheries within a group which looked seamless from outside. The divisions of the basis of school of thought within the Sunni sect of Islam, place of birth in Mirpur and belongingness to a particular clan, immigration pattern, back home politics and political affiliation in the UK provided valid levels of analysis.

The thesis thus theorized community formation as a strategic process in the clash and concurrence of political, social, economic and cultural interests, affiliations and loyalties in an array of power relations operational in a community. This dynamic conceptualisation of subject positions provided the support to my theorisation of community as a fluid and strategic positioning of various subjectivities. The members of the community used various labels like black, ethnic, minority, immigrant, non-white Muslim, Pakistani, Kashmiri, Sunnis strategically. This process of subjectification was not fixed but a dynamic positioning to forge a shared feeling, promote a worldview, organize communal events and engage in debates. And in this flux of positions, Radio Ramzan provided a consistent backdrop linking together the social, cultural, political and spiritual aspects of life. The experiences gained and the lessons learnt from the study of Radio Ramzan in general and the HEAP project in particular require further research to explore the dynamic relationship between place, spirituality and media. Such research is most needed within the 'deprived pockets' of the affluent West where many people because of their status, faith, colour and the area they live in, remain tangled in a vicious circle of disadvantage and discrimination.

This study has made a humble effort in this direction by offering fresh insights in foregrounding the worldviews of marginalized communities living in the back streets of the West. The study has tried to remove the barriers between the theory and practice by practicing theory and theorizing practice simultaneously while the Radio Ramzan was on air. This way the experiences from the inner city found echo in the corridors of the academy, and it is hoped that these experiences will make a contribution in the way the social policies are developed, implemented and evaluated.

As we come to know more about the causes and consequences of the global spread of Covid-19 pandemic, social and economic inequalities emerge as implacable reasons for the uneven impact of this pandemic on disadvantaged and marginalized communities across the world. Disparities due to gender, age, ethnicity, economic status often lead to increased health risks, and Covid-19 revealed these inconsistencies as lack of access to resources, services and culturally appropriate care along with pre-existing barriers increased the vulnerabilities and impacted such groups the most. These revelations indicate the asymmetric power that stifles the voice and deprives people of agency to validate their experiential and contextual knowledge in promoting their own health and wellbeing. The presence and participation of marginalized communities is indispensable for any intervention to develop intercultural approaches in addressing inequalities in health and promoting a more inclusive health education agenda. The lessons learnt from Radio Ramzan and the Health Awareness Project as a pertinent case study to legitimize the marginalized voices in health promotion is very relevant to the current debate on how to address the health inequalities and promote a more equitable health agenda.

Bibliography

Abbas, T. (2005). *Muslim Britain: Communities under pressure*. Zed Books.
Acheson, D. (1998). *Independent inquiry into inequalities in health*. HMSO.
Adams, D. (1995a). *Health issues of women of colour: A cultural diversity perspective*. Sage.
Adams, J. (1995b). *Risk*. University College London.
Afhkami, M. (1999). Gender apartheid, cultural relativism and women's human rights in Muslim societies. In C. W. Howland (Ed.), *Religious fundamentalisms and the human rights of women* (pp. 67–77). St. Martin's Press.
Ahmad, W. (Ed.). (1993). *'Race' and health in contemporary Britain*. Open University.
Ahmad, F. (2003). Still in 'In Progress?' – Methodological dilemmas, tensions and contradictions in theorizing South Asian Muslim Women. In N. Puwar & P. Raghuram (Eds.), *South Asian women in the diaspora* (pp. 43–66). Berg.
Ahmad, F., Modood, T., & Lissenburgh, S. (2003). *South Asian women and employment in Britain: The interaction of gender and ethnicity*. Policy Studies Institute.
Alam C., Masudul., & Mohammad A. N. (1992). A critical examination of the concept of Islamization of knowledge in contemporary times. *Humanomics, 8*(3), 60–107. https://doi.org/10.1108/eb006133.
Al-Faruqi, I. R. (1982). *Islamization of knowledge: The problem, principle, and workplan*. Herndon, VA: IIIT.
Amit, V., & Rapport, N. (2002). *The trouble with community: Anthropological reflections on movement, identity, and collectivity*. Pluto Press.
Andermahr, S., Lovel, T., & Wolkowitz, C. (1997). *A concise glossary of feminist theory*. Arnold.
Anderson, J. (2000). Gender, race, poverty, health and discourses of health reform in the context of globalization: A post-colonial feminist perspective in policy research. *Nursing Inquiry, 7*(4), 220–229.
Anthias, F., & Yuval-Davis, N. (1992). *Racialised boundaries, race, nation, gender, colour and class and the anti-racist struggle*. Routledge.
Anwar, M. (1979). *The myth of return: Pakistanis in Britain*. Heinemann Educational.
Anwar, M. (1985). *Pakistanis in the UK*. New Century.
Anwar, M. (1991). Ethnic minorities|| representation: Voting and electoral politics in Britain, and the role of leaders. In P. Werbner & M. Anwar (Eds.), *Black and ethnic leaderships in Britain: The cultural dimensions of political action* (pp. 41–42). Routledge.
Appadurai, A. (2004). The capacity to aspire: Culture and the terms of recognition. In V. Rao & M. Walton (Eds.), *Culture and public action*. Stanford University Press.
Apter, D. E. (1965). *The Politics of Modernization*. Chicago: University of Chicago Press.

F. Malik, *Addressing Health Inequalities through Community Media*,
https://doi.org/10.1007/978-3-031-35237-9

Atkinson, R., & Davoudi, S. (2000). The concept of social exclusion in the European Union: Context, development and possibilities. *Journal of Common Market Studies, 38*(3), 427–448.

Atton, C. (2001, May 24). Approaching alternative media: Theory and methodology. Paper presented to ICA pre-conference *Our Media, Not Theirs*.

Atton, C., & Couldry, N. (2002). *Alternative media,* introduction (Special Issue on Alternative Media). *Media, Culture and Society, 25*(5), 625–645. Sage.

Bacal, A. (1991). *Ethnicity in social sciences: A view and review of the literature on ethnicity, reprint paper on ethnic relation*. Centre for Research in Ethnic Relation, University of Warwick.

Bagguley, P., & Hussain, Y. (2003). Conflict and cohesion: constructions of 'community' around the 2001 'riots'. In *Communities Conference* (18–20 September 2003).

Balarajan, R. (1991). Ethnic differences in mortality from Ischaemic heart disease and cerebrovascular disease in England and Wales. *British Medical Journal, 302*, 560–564.

Balarajan, R., & Raleigh, V. S. (1995). *Ethnicity and health in England*. HMSO.

Ballard, R. (1991). Azad Kashmir: The view from Mirpur. In *Economic and Political Weekly*, Bombay, pp. 513–517.

Ballard, R. (Ed.). (1994). *Desh Pardesh: The South Asian presence in Britain*. Hurst and Company.

Ballard, R. (2002). Race, culture and ethnicity. In M. Holborn (Ed.), *New developments in sociology*. The Causeway Press.

Bambra, C., Lynch, J., Smith, K. E., & Pickett, K. (2021). Pale rider: Pandemic inequalities. In *The unequal pandemic: Covid-19 and health inequalities* (1st ed., pp. 13–34). Bristol University Press. https://doi.org/10.2307/j.ctv1qp9gnf.9

Banton, M. (1997). *Ethnic and racial consciousness* (2nd ed.). Longman.

Banton, M. (2000). Ethnic conflict. *Sociology, 34*, 481–498.

Banuri, T. (1990). Development and the politics of knowledge: A critical interpretation of the social role of modernisation theories in the development of the third world. In F. A. Marglin & S. A. Marglin (Eds.), *Dominating knowledge: Development, culture and resistance* (Vol. 29-72). Clarendon Press.

Barlow, W. (1988). Community radio in the US: The struggle for a democratic medium. *Media, Culture and Society, 19*, 81–105.

Barrera, M. (1979). *Race and class in the Southwest: A theory of racial inequality*. University of Notre Dame Press.

Barrett, M. (1991). *The politics of truth: From Marx to Foucault*. Polity.

Barth, F. (Ed.). (1969). *Ethnic groups and boundaries: The social organization of culture difference*. Little, Brown.

Barton, M. (2005). Race, gender, class and the theology of empowerment: An Indian perspective. In U. King & T. Beattie (Eds.), *Gender, religion and diversity cross-cultural perspectives* (pp. P225–P237). Continuum International Publishing.

Bastian, S., & Bastian, N. (Eds.). (1996). *Assessing participation: A debate from South Asia*. Konark Publishers.

Bauman, Z. (2000). *Liquid modernity*. Polity.

Bauman, Z. (2001). *Seeking safety in an insecure world*. Polity Press.

Becker, S., & Bryman, A. (Eds.). (2004). *Understanding research for social policy and practice: Themes, methods and approaches* (p. 423). Bristol.

Bellah, R. N. (1965). *Epilogue: Religion and progress in modern Asia*. New York: Free Press.

Beltran, L. (1993). *The quest for democracy in communication: Outstanding Latin American experiences*. Agricultural Communications Documentation Centre.

Benhabib, S. (1995). From identity politics to social feminism: A plea for the nineties. *Philosophy of Education*, 22–36.

Bennett, W. L. (2003). New media power: The internet and global activism. In N. Couldry & J. Curran (Eds.), *Contesting media power: Alternative media in a networked world*. Rowman & Littlefield Publishers.

Berghman, J. (1997). Western Europe: Current Practice and Trends. In D. Hirsch (Ed.), *Social protection and inclusion: European challenges for the United Kingdom*. York: J. Rowntree Foundation.

Bhandari, S., & Mills, R. (2003). *Dynamics of economic well-being: Health Insurance 1996–1999*, Current Population Reports. U.S. Census Bureau.

Bjorkgren, M. (2004). *Liberation theology and feminist theology: Similarities and differences* (Vol. 1, pp. 34–36). Theology and Liberation.

Booth, J. (1980). *A different animal: Local radio and the community*. Independent Broadcasting Authority.

Borda, O. F. (1979). Investigating reality in order to transform it: The Colombian experience. *Dialectical Anthropology, 4*(1), 33–55. https://doi.org/10.1007/bf00417683

Bordenave, J. (1980). *Participation in communication systems for development*. Unpublished paper.

Bordenave, J., & Diaz, E. (1977). *Communication and rural development*. United Nations Educational, Scientific and Cultural Organisation (UNESCO).

Bourdieu, P. (1977). *Outline of a theory of practice*. Cambridge University Press.

Bourdieu, P. (1986). The forms of capital. In J.G. Richardson (Ed.), *Handbook for theory and research for the sociology of education* (pp. 241–258).

Bowring, F. (2000). Social exclusion: Limitations of the debate. *Critical Social Policy, 20*, 307–330.

Boyle, J. S. (1994). Styles of ethnography. In J. Morse (Ed.), *Critical issues in qualitative research methods*. Sage.

Brah, A. (1992). Difference, diversity and differentiation. In J. Donald & A. Rattansi (Eds.), *'Race', culture and difference* (pp. 126–145). Sage Publications.

Brah, A. (1996). *Cartographies of diaspora. Contesting identities*. Routledge.

Brah, A. (2002). Global mobilities, local predicaments: Globalization and the critical imagination. *Feminist Review, 70*(4), 30–45.

Braidotti, R., Charkiewicz, E., Huslet, S., & Wieringa, S. (1994). *Women, the environment and sustainable development*. Zed Books.

Braveman, P. (2016). Health difference, disparity, inequality, or inequity—What difference does it make what we call it?: An approach to conceptualizing and measuring health inequalities and health equity. In M. Buchbinder, M. Rivkin-Fish, & R. L. Walker (Eds.), *Understanding health inequalities and justice: New conversations across the disciplines* (pp. 33–63). University of North Carolina Press.

Brecht, B. (1983). Radio as a means of communication: A talk on the function of radio. In A. Mattelart & S. Siegelaub (Eds.), *Communication and class struggle: Liberation, socialism* (pp. 169–171). International General.

Brewer, J. (2000). *Ethnography*. Open University Press.

British Heart Foundation (BHF). (2000). *South Asians and Heart Disease*. Available: http://www.bhsoc.org/bhf_factfiles/bhs_factfile_april_2000.pdf. Last accessed March 2002

Brunskell, H. (1998). Feminist methodology. In C. Seale (Ed.), *researching society and culture*. Sage.

Bunton, R. (1992). More than a woolly jumper: Health promotion as social regulation. *Critical Public Health, 3*(2), 4–11.

Burchardt, T., Le Grand, J., & Piachaud, D. (2002). Introduction. In J. Hills, J. Le Grand, & D. Piachaud (Eds.), *Understanding social exclusion* (pp. 1–12). Oxford University Press.

Byrne, B., Claire A., Omar K., James N., & William S. (Eds.). (2020). *Ethnicity and race in the UK: State of the nation* (1st ed). Bristol University Press. https://doi.org/10.2307/j.ctv14t47tm.

Byrne, D. (1999). *Social exclusion*. Open University Press.

Callaway, H. (1992). Ethnography and experience: Gender implications in fieldwork and texts. In J. Okely & H. Callways (Eds.), *Anthropology and autobiography* (pp. 29-49). New York, NY: Routledge.

Campbell, C. (2001). Social capital and health: Contextualising health promotion within local community networks. In: S. Baron, J. Field, & V. Bahl (Eds.), *Sociology of Health Illness, 17*(3), 418–429.

Campbell, C., & Carl, M. (2003). Social capital, local community participation and the construction of Pakistani identities in England: Implications for health inequalities policies. *Journal of Health Psychology, 8*(2), 247–262. https://doi.org/10.1177/1359105303008002668
Cantle, T. (2001). *Community cohesion: A report of the independent review team.* Home Office.
Capra, F. (1982). *The turning point*. London: Fontana/Flamingo.
Carby, H. (1982). White woman listen! Feminism and the boundaries of sisterhood. In *The Empire Strikes Back* (pp. 212–235). Centre for Contemporary Cultural Studies.
Castells, M. (1983). *The city and the grassroots*. Berkeley and Los Angeles, University of California Press.
Chambers, R. (1992). Rural *appraisal: Rapid, relaxed and participatory*, Institute for Development Studies Discussion paper No. 311. Brighton.
Chambers, R. (1997). *Whose reality counts?* Intermediate Technology Publications.
Chambers, R. (2001). Rural appraisal: Rapid, relaxed and participatory. In A. Mukherjee & R. Chambers (Eds.), *Participatory rural appraisal: Methods and applications in rural planning* (2nd ed., pp. 1–86). Concept Publishing.
Chaturvedi, N., & Fuller, J. H. (1995). Mortality risk by body weight and weight change in people with NIDDM: The WHO Multinational Study of Vascular Disease. *Diabetes Care, 18*, 766–774.
Chouhan, K., & Nazroo, J. (2020). Health inequalities. In B. Byrne, C. Alexander, O. Khan, J. Nazro, & W. Shankley (Eds.), *Ethnicity and race in the UK: State of the nation* (1st ed., pp. 73–92). Bristol University Press. https://doi.org/10.2307/j.ctv14t47tm.10
Clarke, A. (1992). Citizens, markets and consumers: A post welfare state view of leisure. In J. Sugden & C. Knox (Eds.), *Leisure in the 1990s: Rolling back the Welfare State* (Publication No. 46) (pp. 109–120). LSA Publications.
Clarke, J. (2000). *New managerialism, new welfare?* London: Sage Publications.
Clarke, J. (2005). New labour's citizens: Activated, empowered, responsiblised, abandoned? *Citizenship Studies, 2*(25), 447–463.
Coid, J. W., Kahtan, N., & Gault, S. (2000). Ethnic differences in admissions to secure forensic psychiatry services. *British Journal of Psychiatry, 177*, 241–247.
Coker, N. (2002). *Racism in medicine: An agenda for change*. King's Fund.
Coleman, J. (1988). Organizations and institutions: Sociological and economic approaches to the analysis of social structure. *The American Journal of Sociology, 94*, S95–S120.
Collins, H. P. (1990). *Black feminist thought: Knowledge, consciousness, and the politics of empowerment*. Routledge.
Collins, P. H. (1991). Learning from the outsider within: The sociological significance of Black feminist thought. In M. M. Fonow & J. A. Cook (Eds.), *Beyond methodology: Feminist scholarship as lived research* (pp. 35–39). Indiana University Press.
Cooke, B., & Kothari, U. (2003). Participation: The New Tyranny. http://www.lst-iiep.iiep-unesco.org/cgi-bin/wwwi32.exe/[in=epidoc1.in]/?t2000=012096/(100). 23. 10.1016/S0738-0593(02)00022-6.
Corbridge, S. (1998). 'Beneath the pavement only soil': The poverty of post-development. *Journal of Development Studies, 34*(6), 138–148. https://doi.org/10.1080/00220389808422549.
Couldry, N. (1999). "Disrupting the Media Frame at Greenham Common: A New Chapter in the History of Mediations?" *Media, Culture & Society 21*(3): 337–58. https://doi.org/10.1177/016344399021003003.
Couldry, N. (2001). The umbrella man: Crossing a landscape of speech and silence. *European Journal of Cultural Studies, 4*(2), 131–153.
Couldry, N. (2003). *Media rituals: A critical approach*. Routledge.
Cowen, M., & Shenton, N. (1995). The invention of development. In J. Crush (Ed.), (pp. 27–43). Routledge.
Cox, O. C. (1948/1970). *Caste, class and race: A study in social dynamics*. Monthly Review (Modern Reader).
Cox, E. (1995). *A truly civil society*. Boyer Lectures, Australian Broadcasting Corporation.
Craig, G., Taylor, M., Szanto, C., & Wilkinson, M. (1999). *Developing 'local compacts' between local government and the voluntary sector*. Joseph Rowntree Foundation.

Crush, J. S. (1995). *Power of development*. Routledge.
Dagron, A. G. (2001). *Making waves: Stories of participatory communication for social change*. The Rockefeller Foundation.
Dallmayr, F. (1993). *Modernisation and postmodernisation: Theoretical comments on India*. Available: http://kellogg.nd.edu/publications/workingpapers/WPS/195.pdf. Last accessed 22 June 2003.
Davies, B. (1993). *Shards of glass: Children reading and writing beyond gendered identities*. Allen & Unwin.
Davies, M. W. (2002). *Wilful imaginings*. Available: http://www.newint.org/features/2002/05/01/wilful-imaginings/. Last accessed 02 Dec 2002.
Davies, J., & Macdonald, G. (1998). *Quality, evidence, and effectiveness in health promotion: Striving for certainties*. Routledge.
Davis, C. (1993). *After poststructuralism: Reading, stories and theory*. Routledge.
Day, G., & Murdoch, J. (1993). Locality and community: Coming to terms with place. *Sociological Review, 41*(1), 82–111.
Dayha, B. (1974). The nature of Pakistani ethnicity in industrial cities in Britain. In A. Cohen (Ed.), *Cohen, A: Urban ethnicity* (pp. 77–113). Tavistock.
Denny, F. M. (1985). *An introduction to Islam*. Macmillan.
Department of Health. (1988). *Primary health care: An agenda for discussion*. HMSO.
Department of Health. (1991). *Health of the nation*. DoH.
Department of Health. (1998). *Our Healthier Nation: A contract for health*. HMSO.
Department of Health. (1999). *Reducing Health Inequalities: An action report*. DoH.
Department of Health. (2000). Department of Health, and Sir Donald Acheson, Independent Inquiry into inequalities in Health Report.
Department of Health, & Sir Donald Acheson. (1998). *Independent inquiry into inequalities in health report*.
Department of Transport and Regions. (2000). *Indices of deprivation*. DETR.
Desai, R. (1963). *Indian immigrants in Britain London*. London Oxford University Press and The Institute for Race Relations.
Dewey, J. (1938). *Experience and education*. Collier Books.
Downing, J. (1984). *Radical media: The political experience of alternative communication*. South End Press.
Downing, J. (2001). *Radical media: Rebellious communication and social movements*. Sage.
Downing, J. (2003). The independent media center movement and the Anarchist socialist tradition. In N. Couldry & J. Curran (Eds.). Contesting Media.
Eade, J. (1989). *The politics of community*. Gower Publishing.
EEC. (1995). On specific community action to combat poverty (Council Decision of 19 December 1984). *Official Journal of the EEC 85/8/EEC*, 2–24.
Engineer, A. (2000). *Muhammad (PBUH) as liberator: Islam and modern age*. http://ecumene.org/Iis/csss37.htm. Date accessed 30 July 2002.
Engineer, A. (2007). *Islam in contemporary world*. Sterling.
England, P. (1993). *Theory on gender / feminism on theory*. Aldine.
Enzensberger, H. M. (1974). *The consciousness industry: On literature, politics and the media*. Seabury.
Erens, B., Primtesta, P., & Prior, G. (Eds.). (1999). *Health survey for England: The health of minority ethnic groups*. London.
Esak, F. (1997). *Quran, liberation and pluralism: An Islamic perspective of interreligious solidarity against oppression*. One World Publications.
Escobar, A. (1988). Power and visibility: Development and the intervention and management of the "Third World". *Cultural Anthropology, 3*(4), 428–453.
Escobar, A. (1992). Planning. In W. Sachs (Ed.), *The development dictionary: A guide to knowledge as power*. Zed Books.
Escobar, A. (1995a). Imagining a post-development era. In J. Crush (Ed.), *Power of development*. Routledge.

Escobar, A. (1995b). *Encountering development: The making and unmaking of the "Third World"*. Princeton University.
Escobar, A. (1997). Anthropology and development. *International Social Science Journal, 49*(4), 497–516.
Esteva, G. (1987). Regenerating people's space. *Alternatives, 12*, 125–152.
Esteva, G. (1992). Development. In W. Sachs (Ed.), *The development dictionary: A guide to knowledge as power* (pp. 6–25). ZED.
Fals-Borda, O., & Rahman, M. (1991). *Action and knowledge: Breaking the monopoly with participatory action-research.* The Apex Press.
Farnell, R. (2001). Faith communities, regeneration and social exclusion: Developing a research agenda. *Community Development Journal, 36*(4).
Farnell, R., Lund, S., Furbey, R., Lawless, P., Wishart, B., & Else, P. (1994). *Hope in the city? The local impact of the Church Urban Fund.* Centre for Regional Economic and Social Research, Sheffield Hallam University.
Farnell, R., Furbey, R., Hills, S., Macy, M., & Mith, G. (2003). *'Faith' in urban regeneration? Engaging faith communities in urban regeneration.* The Policy Press.
Farrow, L. (1974). *Feminism as Anarchism, quiet rumors.* Dark Star.
Fawcett, J. (1984). *Analysis and evaluation of conceptual models of nursing*. Davis.
Fenton, S. (1999). *Ethnicity: Racism, class & culture.* Macmillan.
Fernandes, W., & Tandon, R. (Eds.). (1981). *Participatory research and evaluation: Experiments in research as a process of liberation.* Indian Social Institute.
Fernando, S. (1991). *Mental health, race and culture.* London: Macmillan.
Fernando, S., Egger, G., & Spark, R. (1993). *Health promotion strategies and methods* (Revised Ed.). McGraw Hill.
Finn, J. (1994). The promise of participatory research. *Journal of Progressive Human Services, 5*(2), 25–42.
Fiske, J. (1982). *Introduction to communication studies*. Methuen.
Fleming, M. L., & Parker, E. (Elizabeth Anne), 1945–. (2001). *Health promotion: Principles and practice in the Australian context* / Mary Louise O'Connor-Fleming and Elizabeth Parker. Crows Nest, N.S.W.: Allen & Unwin.
Forrest, R., & Kearns, A. (1999). *Joined-up places?* Joseph Rowntree Foundation.
Foucault, M. (1972). *The archeology of knowledge* (A.M. Sheridan-Smith, Trans.). Tavistock.
Foucault, M. (1979). *Discipline and punish: The birth of the prison* (A. Sheridan, Trans.). Vintage/ Random House.
Foucault, M. (1980). Truth and power. In C. Gordon (Ed.), *Michel Foucault: Power/knowledge, selected interviews and other writings 1972–1977* (pp. 109–133). Harvester Press.
Foucault, M. (1982). The subject and power. Afterword. In H. L. Dreyfus & P. Rabinow (Eds.), *Michel Foucault: Beyond structuralism and hermeneutics* (pp. 208–226). Harvester Press.
Fraser, N. (1995). Politics, culture, and the public sphere: Toward a postmodern conception. In L. J. Nicholson & S. Seidman (Eds.), *Social postmodernism*. Cambridge University Press.
Fraser, N., & Nicholson, L. (1990). Social criticism without philosophy: An encounter between Feminism and Postmodernism. In L. Nicholson (Ed.), *Feminism/ Postmoderinsim*. Routledge.
Fraser, N., & Nicholson, L. (1993). *The politics of community: A feminist analysis of the liberal-communitarian debate*. Harvester Wheatsheaf.
Fredman, S., Alston, P., & Burca, G. (2001). *Discrimination and human rights*. Oxford University Press.
Free, C., & Mckee, M. (1998). Meeting the needs of black and minority ethnic groups. *British Medical Journal, 316*, 380.
Freire, P. (1972). *Pedagogy of the oppressed*. Penguin, London.
Freire, P. (1974). *Education for critical consciousness*. Seabury.
Freire, P. (1985). *The politics of education, culture power and liberation* (D. Macedo, Trans.). Bergin & Garvey.

Friberg, M., & Hettene, B. (1985). The greening of the world - Towards a non deterministic model of global processes. In *Development as social transformation* (pp. 204–270). Hodder and Stoughton.

Furbey, R. (1999). Urban regeneration: Reflections on a metaphor. *Critical Social Policy, 19*(4), 419–455.

Ganguly, S. (1997). *The crisis in Kashmir: Portents of war, hopes of peace*. Cambridge: Cambridge University Press.

Genzuk, M. (2003). *A synthesis of ethnographic research* (Occasional Papers Series). Center for Multilingual, Multicultural Research (Eds.). Center for Multilingual, Multicultural Research, Rossier School of Education, University of Southern California.

Giddens, A. (1976). *New rules of sociological method*. Basic Books.

Giddens, A. (1987). *The nation-state and violence*. University of California Press.

Giddens, A. (1991). *The consequences of modernity*. Stanford University Press.

Gilroy, P. (1982). *The empire strikes back - Race and racism in 70s Britain*. Centre for Contemporary Cultural Studies.

Goldberg, D. (1999). Cultural aspects of mental disorder in primary care. In D. Bhugra & V. Bahal (Eds.), *An agenda for mental health* (pp. 23–28). Gaskell.

Golding, P. (1974). Media role in national development: Critique of a theoretical orthodoxy. *Journal of Communication, 24*(3), 39–53.

Graham, H. (2004). Social determinants and their unequal distribution: Clarifying policy understandings. *Milbank Q., 82*(1), 101–124. https://doi.org/10.1111/j.0887-378x.2004.00303.x. PMID: 15016245; PMCID: PMC2690205

Gramsci, A. (1971). *Selections from the prison notebooks*. International Publishers.

Greener, I. (1999). *Shifting the paradigm: Managerialism in the NHS*. Paper presented to Critical Management Studies Conference, Public Sector Stream, Manchester University (14–16, July 1999).

Greener, I. (2002). Understanding NHS reform: The policy-transfer, social learning, and path-dependency perspectives. *Governance, 15*(2), 161–183.

Groenhout, R. F. (2002). *Philosophy, feminism, and faith*. Indiana University Press.

Gutierrez, G. (1988). *A theology of liberation: History, politics and salvation*. Orbis Books.

Hague, E., Thomas, C., & Willimas, S. (1999). Left out? Observations on the RGSIBG conference on social exclusion and the city. *Area, 31*(3), 293–296.

Haig, B. (1997). Feminist research methodology. In J. P. Keeves (Ed.), *Educational research methodology and measurement* (pp. 297–302). Pergamon.

Hall, S. (1988). *The hard road to renewal: Thatcherism and the crisis of the left*. Verso.

Hall, S. (1991). Old and new identities, old and new ethnicities. In A. D. King (Ed.), *Culture, globalization and the world system: Contemporary conditions for the representation of Identity*. Macmillan.

Hall, S. (1992a). The west and the rest: Discourse and power. In S. Hall & B. Gielben (Eds.), *Chapter six of Formations of modernity* (pp. 276–320). Polity Press.

Hall, S. (1992b). Cultural studies and its theoretical legacies. In L. Grossberg et al. (Eds.), *Cultural studies* (pp. 261–274). Routledge.

Hall, S. (1997). *Representation: Cultural representations and signifying practices*. Sage.

Hall, S., & Jefferson, T. (1977). *Resistance through rituals: Youth subcultures in post-war Britain*. Hutchinson.

Hall, S., Critcher, C., Jefferson, T., Clarke, J., & Roberts, B. (1978). *Policing the crisis*. Macmillan.

Hardill, I., Graham, D. T., & Kofman, E. (2001). *Human geography of the UK: An introduction*. Routledge.

Harding, S. (1991). *Whose science? Whose knowledge? Thinking from women's lives*. Cornell University Press.

Harding, S. (1998). *Is science multicultural? Postcolonialisms, feminisms, and epistemologies*. Indiana University Press.

Harrison, G., Owens, D., Holton, A., Neilson, D., & Boot, D. (1988). A prospective study of severe mental disorder in Afro-Caribbean patients. *Psychological Medicine, 18*(3), 643–657.

Hartley, J. (2000). Radiocracy: Sound and citizenship. *International Journal of Cultural Studies, 3*(2), 153–159.

Harvey, D. (1973). *Social justice and the city*. Edward Arnold.

Harvey, L. (1990). *Critical social research*. Unwin Hyman.

Haw, K. (1998). *Educating Muslim girls: Shifting discourses*. Oxford University Press.

Herman, S., & Chomsky, N. (1988). *Manufacturing consent: The political economy of the mass media*. Pentheaon Books.

Hill, C. P. (2000). *Black feminist thought: Knowledge, consciousness, and the politics of empowerment*. Routledge.

Hoggart, L., Sales, R., Roman, I., & Gunbey, A. (2000). *Turkish speaking mothers in Hackney*. Social Policy Research Centre, Middlesex University.

Hollander, E. (1992). The emergence of small scale media. In N. Jankowski, O. Prehn, & J. Stappers (Eds.), *The people's voice: Local radio and television in Europe*. John Libbey.

Hollander E., & Stappers, J. (1992). Community media and community communication. In J. Jankowski, O. Prehn & J. Stappers (Eds.), *The people's voice: Local radio and television in Europe*. John Libbey.

Hollander, E., Stappers, J., & Jankowski, N. (2002). Community media and community communication. In N. Jankowski & O. Prehn (Eds.), *Community media in the information age*. Hampton Press.

Hollway, W. (1984). Gender difference and the production of subjectivity. In J. Henriques & W. Hooks (Eds.), *Feminist theory: From margin to center* (2nd ed.). South End Press.

Hollway, W., Urwin, C., Venn, L., & Walkerdine, V. (Eds.). (1984). *Changing the subject: Psychology, social regulation and subjectivity* (pp. 227–263). Methuen.

Humphries, B., & Truman, C. (Eds.). (1994). *Re-thinking social research: Anti-discriminatory approaches in research methodology*. Ashgate Publishing.

Huppert, F. A. (2009). A new approach to reducing disorder and improving wellbeing. *Perspectives on Psychological Science, 4*, 108–111.

IISD. (1995). *World Summit for social development*. Available: http://www.iisd.ca/wssd95.html. Last accessed 18 July 2001.

Inkleles, A. (1974). The modernisation of man. In M. Weiner (Ed.), *Modernisation: The dynamics of growth* (pp. 138–150). Free Press.

Jannkowski, N., Prehn, O., & Stappers, J. (1992). *The People's voice: Local radio and knowledge as power* (pp 132–145). Zed Books.

Jayaratne, T., & Stewart, A. (1991). Quantitative and qualitative methods in the social sciences current feminist issues and practical strategies. In *Beyond methodology: Feminist scholarship as lived research*. Indiana University Press.

Jeffery, P. (1976). *Migrants and refugees: Muslim and Christian Pakistani families in Bristol Cambridge*. Cambridge University Press.

Jensen, A. (1969). How much can we boost IQ and scholastic achievement? *Harvard Educational Review, 39*(1), 1–123.

Jensen, A. R. (1973). *Educability and group differences*. Harper and Rowe.

Kabeer, N. (1999). Resources, agency, and achievements: Reflections on the measurement of women's empowerment. *Development and Change, 30*, 435–464. https://doi.org/10.1111/1467-7660.00125

Kamler, B., Maclean, R., Reid, J., & Simpson, A. (1994). *Shaping up nicely: The formation of schoolgirls and schoolboys in the first month of school*. Australian Government Printing.

Karawan, I. (1992). Monarchs, Mullas, and Marshals: Islamic Regimes? *The Annals of the American Academy of Political and Social Science, 524*, 103–119.

Karlsen, S., & Nazroo, J. Y. (2001). Agency and structure: The impact of ethnic identity and racism on the health of ethnic minority people. *Sociology of Health and Illness, 24*(1), 1–20.

Karlsen, S., & Nazroo, J. Y. (2002). Relation between racial discrimination, social class, and health among ethnic minority groups. *American Journal of Public Health, 92*, 624–631.

Katz, C. (1994). Playing the field: Questions of fieldwork in geography. *The Professional Geographer, 46*(1), 67–72.

Kawachi, I., Kennedy, B., Lochner, K., & Prothrow-Stith, D. (1997). Social capital, income inequality, and mortality. *Journal of Public Health, 87*, 1491–1498.

Kawachi, I., Subramanian, S. V., & Almeida-Filho, N. (2002). A glossary for health inequalities. *Journal of Epidemiology and Community Health (1979-), 56*(9), 647–652. http://www.jstor.org/stable/25569791

Kellner, D. (1995). *Media culture: Cultural studies, identity, and politics between the modern and the postmodern*. Routledge.

Kellner, D. (2001). *Critical theory, poststructuralism.* Available: http://www.uta.edu/huma/illuminations/kell7.htm. Last accessed 22 July 2004.

Kempson, E., & Whyley, C. (1999). *Understanding and combating 'financial exclusion'*. JRF.

Kendall, L. (2001). *The future patient*. Institute for Public Policy Research.

Kenneth, R., McLeroy, Barbara L. Norton, Michelle C. Kegler, James N. Burdine, & Ciro V. Sumaya. (2003). Community-Based Interventions. *American Journal of Public Health, 93*, 529–533.

Khan, M. I. (1997). *Experiencing Islam*. New Delhi: Sterling Publishing.

King, D. (1988). Multiple jeopardy, multiple consciousness: The context of a black feminist ideology. *Signs: Journal of Women in Culture and Society, 14*, 42–72.

Knibbe, M., De Vries, M., & Horstman, K. (2017). Engaging cultural resources to promote mental health in Dutch LSES neighborhoods: Study of a community-based participatory media project. *Health Promotion International, 32*(3), 567–576.

Knitter, P. (1987). Toward a liberation theology of religions. In J. Hick & P. Knitter (Eds.), *The myth of Christian uniqueness: Toward a pluralistic theology of religions* (pp. 178–202). Orbis Books.

Kobayashi, A. (1994). Coloring the field: Gender, race, and the politics of fieldwork. *The Professional Geographer, 46*(1), 73–80.

Kothari, R. (1998). *State against democracy: In search of human governance*. Ajanta Publishers.

Kristsman, L. D. 1990. (Michel Foucault politics philosophy culture).

Kumar, J. K. (2000). *Mass communication in India*. Jaico.

Laclau, E. (1994). The impossibility of society. In *Emancipations*. Verso.

Laclau, E., & Mouffe, C. (1985). *Hegemony and socialist strategy: Towards a radical democratic politics*. Verso.

Laird, L. D., Amer, M. M., Barnett, E. D., & Barnes, L. L. (2007). Muslim patients and health disparities in the UK and the US. *Archives of Disease in Childhood, 92*(10), 922–926.

Lamb, A. (2003). *Kashmir: A disputed legacy, 1846–1990*. Karachi: Oxford University Press.

Latham, M. E. (2000). *Modernisation as ideology: American social science and nation building in the Kennedy era*. University of North Carolina Press.

Lather, P. (1991). *Getting smart: Feminist research and pedagogy within the postmodern*. Routledge.

Learmonth, M. (1997). Managerialism and public attitudes towards UK NHS managers. *Journal of Management in Medicine, 11*(4), 214–221. https://doi.org/10.1108/02689239710177314

Leeuw, D., & Hussein, A. (1999). Islamic health promotion and interculturalization. *Health Promotion International, 14*(4), 347–353.

Lerner, D. (1958). *The passing of traditional society: Modernizing the Middle East*. The Free Press.

Levin, J. (1996). How religion influences morbidity and health: Reflections on natural history, salutogenesis and host resistance. *Social Science and Medicine, 43*(5), 849–864.

Levin, J. (2001). *God, faith, and health: Exploring the spirituality-healing connection*. Wiley.

Levin, J. S., & Schiller, P. L. (1987). Is there a religious factor in health? *Journal of Religion and Health, 26*, 9–36.

Levitas, R. (1998). *The inclusive society? Social exclusion and new labour*. Macmillan.

Levitas, R. (1999). Defining and measuring social exclusion: A critical overview of current proposals. *Radical Statistics, 71*, 10–27.

Levitas, R., & Gordon, D. (2000). *Poverty and social exclusion in Britain*. Joseph Rowntree Foundation.

Lewis, O. (1959). *Five families*. Basic Books.
Lewis, P. (1994). *Islamic Britain: Religion, politics and identity among British Muslims*. I. B. Tauris.
Lewis, P. (2003). *Alternative media; Linking the global and local*. UNESCO.
Lewis, P., & Booth, J. (1989). *The invisible medium: Public, commercial and community radio*. Macmillan Education.
Lincoln, Y. S. (Ed.). *Handbook of qualitative research*. Sage.
Lloyd, D. (1999). *Introduction to Topoi*. http://humanities.uchicago.edu/orgs/institute/mellon/Lloyd.pdf. Date accessed 15 July 20002.
Lloyd, P., & Moodley, P. (1992). Psychotropic medication and ethnicity: An inpatient survey. *Social Psychiatry and Psychiatric Epidemiology, 27*, 95–101.
Lomas, J. (1998). Social capital and health implications for public health and epidemiology. *Social Science and Medicine, 47*(9), 1181–1188.
Lowe, K. (1998). Gender maps. In N. Yelland (Ed.), *Gender in early childhood*. Routledge.
Luke, C., & Gore, J. (Eds.). (1992). *Feminisms and critical pedagogy*. Routledge.
Lukes, S. (1974). *Power: A radical view*. Macmillan.
Lukes, S. (1977). Power and structure. In S. Lukes (Ed.), *Essays in social theory*. Macmillan.
Lupton, D. (1995). *The imperative of health: Public health and the regulated body*. London: SAGE Publications.
Macpherson Report. (1999). Office, Home. "The Stephen Lawrence Inquiry." GOV.UK, February 24, 1999. https://www.gov.uk/government/publications/the-stephen-lawrence-inquiry.
Madanipour, A., Cars, G., & Allen, J. (Eds.). (1998). *Social exclusion in European cities: Processes, experiences, and responses*. Jessica Kingsley.
Madge, C., Raghuram, P., Skelton, T., Willis, K., & Williams, J. (1997). Feminist methodologies: Politics, practice and power. In Women and Geography Study Group (WGSG) (Ed.), *Feminist geography: Explorations in diversity and difference* (pp. 86–111). Prentice Hall.
Marmot, M., & Siegrist, J. (Ed.). (2004). Health inequalities and the psychosocial environment [Editorial]. *Social Science & Medicine, 58*(8), 14–61. https://doi.org/10.1016/S0277-9536(03)00348-4
Marmot, M., & Wilkinson, R. G. (1999). *Social determineants of health*. Oxford: Oxford University Press.
Marsh, A., & David, M. (1998). *Housing and public policy: Citizenship, choice, and control*. Buckingham England: Open University Press.
Massey, D. (1991). A global sense of place. *Marxism Today, June*, 24–29.
Maududi, M. (1988). *Towards understanding the Quran* (Z.I. Ansari, Trans. and Ed.). The Islamic Foundation.
Mayo, M., & Craig, G. (1995). Community participation and empowerment: The human face of structural adjustment or tools for democratic transformation? In G. Craig & M. Mayo (Eds.), *Community empowerment: A reader in participation and development* (pp. 1–11). Zed Books.
MCB. (2003). *Increasing health awareness*. Available: http://www.mcb.org.uk/features/features.php?ann_id=149. Last accessed 14 May 2004.
McCartney, G., Popham, F., McMaster, R., & Cumbers, A. (2019, July). Defining health and health inequalities. *Public Health, 172*, 22–30. https://doi.org/10.1016/j.puhe.2019.03.023. Epub 2019 May 31. PMID: 31154234; PMCID: PMC6558275
Mckenzie, K. (2003). Racism and health. *British Medical Journal, 326*(7380), 65–66.
Mclean, C., & Campbell, C. (2001). *Mental health advocacy and the Pakistani Kashmiri community in Luton*. Luton Health Action Zone.
Mcquail, D. (1994). *Mass communication theory: An introduction* (3rd ed.). Sage.
Mcquail, D. (2000). *Mass communication theory* (4th ed.). Sage.
Mead, G. H. (1934). Mind, self, & society from the standpoint of a social behaviorist. In C. W. Morris (Ed.), *pp* (pp. 68–90). University of Chicago Press.
Melanchthon, M. (2005). Indian Dalit women and the bible: Hermeneutical and methodological reflection. In U. King & T. Beattie (Eds.), *Gender, religion and diversity cross-cultural perspectives* (pp. 212–224). Continum International Publishing.

Melkote, S., & Steeves, H. (2001). *Communication for development in the "Third World": Theory and practice for empowerment* (2nd ed.). Sage.

Mies, M. (1999). Towards a methodology for feminist research. In A. Brayman & J. Smith (Eds.) 1991, *A methodology for twenty-first century sociology. Social Forces* (Vol. 70, pp. 1–17).

Mocroft, I., Pharoah, C and Romney-Alexander, D. 1999. Healthy relationships: A survey of London health authorities' and trusts' support to the voluntary sector.

Modood, T. (1992). *Not easy being British: Colour, culture and citizenship*. Runnymede Trust and Trentham Books.

Modood, T. (1997). Introduction: The politics of multiculturalism in the New Europe. In T. Modood & P. Werbner (Eds.), *The politics of multiculturalism* (p. 1524). Zed.

Modood, T. (1998). Anti-essentialism, multiculturalism and the 'recognition' of religious groups. *Journal of Political Philosophy, 6*(4), 378–399. https://doi.org/10.1111/1467-9760.00060.

Modood, T. (2004). *Defined by some distinctly hyphenated Britishness*. Available: http://www.timeshighereducation.co.uk/story.asp?storycode=190960. Last accessed October 2004.

Modood, T., & Ahmad, F. (2007). British Muslim perspectives on multiculturalism. *Theory Culture Society, 24*, 187–213.

Modood, T., Beishon, S., & Virdee, S. (1994). *Changing ethnic identities*. Policy Studies Institute.

Modood, T., Berthoud, R., Lakey, J., Nazroo, J., Smith, P., Virdee, S., & Beishon, S. (1997). *Ethnic minorities in Britain: Diversity and disadvantage*. Policy Studies Institute.

Mohanty, C. T. (1988). Under Western eyes: Feminist scholarships and colonial discourses. *Feminist Review, 30*, 61–88.

Mohanty, C. T. (2002). Under Western eyes: Feminist scholarship and colonial discourses. In H. Y. Jung (Ed.), *Comparative political culture in the age of globalization: An introductory anthology* (pp. 159–188). Lexington Books.

Mohanty, C. T. (2003). *Feminism without borders: Decolonizing theory, practicing solidarity*. Duke University Press.

Moon, G., & Powell, M. (2001). Health Action Zones: The third way of a new area-based policy? *Health & Social Care in the Community, 9*(1), 43–50.

Moynihan, D. P. (1965). *Employment, income, and the ordeal of the Negro family*. Indianapolis: Bobbs-Merrill Co.

Musgrave, P. with Chester, M., Farrands, M. et al. (1998). Flourishing communities: Engaging church communities with government in the New Deal for communities. Church Urban Fund, Church Action on Poverty and Churches Community Work Alliance, London.

Munoz, G. (2002). *Islam's women under Western eyes*. Available: http://www.opendemocracy.net/faith-europe_islam/article_498.jsp. Last accessed 15 July 2005.

Murad, A. H. (1998). *Book review of Farid Esack's the Quran, liberation and plurallism*. Available: http://www.masud.co.UK/Islam/ahm/esack.htm. Last accessed 13 October 2002.

Muslim Hands, UK. (2001). Available: http://www.muslimhands.org/en/gb/about_mh/our_history/. Last accessed March 2002.

Nagar, N., & Raju, S. (2003). *Women, NGOS and the contradictions of empowerment and disempowerment: A conversation*. Blackwell Publishing.

Nandy, A. (1992). State. In W. Sachs (Ed.), *Development dictionary* (pp. 264–274). Zed Book.

Narayan, U. (1989). The project of feminist epistemology. In S. Bordo & A. Jaggar (Eds.), *Gender/body/knowledge: Feminist reconstructions of being and knowing* (pp. 256–272). Rutgers University Press.

Navarro, V. (2002). Politics, power, and quality of life: A critique of social capital. *International Journal of Health Services, 32*(3), 423–432.

Nazroo, J. (1997). *The health of Britain's ethnic minorities*. Policy Studies Institute.

Nazroo, J. (1998). Genetic, cultural or socioeconomic vulnerability? Explaining ethnic inequalities in health. *Sociology of Health & Illness, 20*(5), 710–730.

Nazroo, J. (2000). Nottingham Social Action Research project (SARP) Baseline Survey. *Findings from a survey of adults aged 16 and over in two areas of Nottingham*. Division of public health medicine and Epidemiology, University of Nottingham.

Nazroo, J. Y. (2001). *Ethnicity, class and health.* Policy Studies Institute.

Nazroo, J. Y. (2003). The structuring of ethnic inequalities in health: Economic position, racial discrimination, and racism. *Am J Public Health, 93*(2), 277–284. https://doi.org/10.2105/ajph.93.2.277. PMID: 12554585; PMCID: PMC1447729.

Nazroo, J., & Karlsen, S. (2001). *Ethnic inequalities in health: Social class, racism and identity.* Lancaster University.

Negrine, R. (1989). *Politics and mass media in Britain.* Routledge.

Nelson, N., & Wright, S. (1995). Participation and power. In N. Nelson & S. Wright (Eds.), *Power and participatory development: Theory and practice* (pp. 1–18). Intermediate Technology Publications.

Nerwal, H. (1997). *A study into the health needs of the Mirpuri Punjabi speaking population of Nottingham,* Unpublished report. Nottingham Health Authority.

Newby, H. (1980). *Green and pleasant land?: Social change in rural England.* Penguin.

Newby, H., & Bell, C. (1981). *Community studies: An introduction to the sociology of the local community.* Unwin University Books.

Nielsen, J. (ed.), (1990). *Feminist research methods.* Boulder, Col.: Westview.

Nielsen, L., & Albertsen, A. (2023). Pandemic justice: Fairness, social inequality and COVID-19 healthcare priority-setting. *Journal of Medical Ethics, 49*, 283–287.

O'Brien, D., Wilkes, J., de Haan, A., & Maxwell, S. (1997). Poverty and social exclusion in North and South (IDS Working Paper No. 55). *Institute of development studies and poverty research unit*, University of Sussex. Indianapolis: Bobbs-Merrill Co.

Ocloo, J. (2021). Silenced voices, unequal impact: Addressing health inequities and discrimination in co-producing health and care during the pandemic and beyond. In J. Ocloo, P. Beresford, M. Farr, G. Hickey, M. Kaur, D. Tembo, & O. Williams (Eds.), *Covid-19 and co-production in health and social care research, policy, and practice: Volume 1: The Challenges and necessity of co-production.*

Office, Home. (1999, February 24). The Stephen Lawrence Inquiry. *GOV.UK.* https://www.gov.uk/government/publications/the-stephen-lawrence-inquiry.

ONS. (2003). *Census 2001 - Ethnicity and religion in England and Wales.* Available: http://www.statistics.gov.uk/census2001/profiles/commentaries/ethnicity.asp. Last accessed December 03.

ONS. (2021). https://www.ons.gov.uk/peoplepopulationandcommunity/healthandsocialcare/healthandwellbeing/bulletins/healthinengland/2015to2021

Owen, D. W. (1994). South Asian People in Great Britain: Social and economic circumstances, *National Ethnic Minority Data Archive 1991 Census Statistical Paper no. 7,* Centre for Research in Ethnic Relations, University of Warwick.

Park, P. (1993). What is participatory research? A theoretical and methodological perspective. In P. Park, M. Brydon-Miller, B. Hall, & T. Jackson (Eds.), *Voices of change* (pp. 1–19). Bergin & Garvey.

Partridge, S. (1982). *Not the BBC/IBA: The case for community radio.* Comedia.

Penna, S. (2004). Policy contexts of social work in Britain: The wider implications of 'New' labour and the 'New legal regime'. *Social Work & Society, 1*(1), 1–21.

Phillips, D. (1998). Black minority ethnic concentration, segregation and dispersal in Britain. *Urban Studies, 35*(10), 1681–1702. https://doi.org/10.1080/0042098984105.

Pierson, J. (2004). *Tackling social exclusion.* Routledge.

Powell, A. (2002). *Mental health and spirituality.* www.rcpsych.ac.uk/college/sig/spirit/publications/index.htm. Date accessed 10 Jan 2003.

Powell, R. M., & Joanne, N. (2021). Addressing risk factors among parents with serious mental illness: Commentary on Ostrow Et Al. *Psychiatric Services* (Washington D.c.) 466–467. https://doi.org/10.1176/appi.ps.202000790

Power, A., & Wilson, W. J. (2000). *Social exclusion and the future of cities,* Case paper, 35. LSE.

Prehn, O. (1992). From small scale utopianism to large scale pragmatism. Trends and prospects for community orientated local radio and television'. In J. Jankowski, O. Prehn, & J. Stappers (Eds.), *The people's voice: Local radio and television in Europe.* John Libbey Press.

Pryce, K. (1979). *Endless pressure*. Classical.

Putnam, L. L., & Mumby, D. K. (1993). Organizations, emotion, and the myth of rationality. In S. Fineman (Ed.), *Emotion in organizations* (pp. 36–57). Sage.

Purdy, M., & Banks, D. (Eds.). (1999). *Health and exclusion: Policy and practice in health provisions*. Routledge.

Raghuram, P. (1999). Religion and development. In T. Skelton & T. Allen (Eds.), *Culture and global change* (pp. 234–246). Routledge.

Raghuram, P. (2007). Interrogating the language of integration: The case of IRNS. *Journal of Clinical of Clinical Nursing, 16*(12), 2246–2251.

Raghuram, P., Madge, C., & Skelton, T. (1998). Feminist methodologies and student research projects. *Journal of Geography in Higher Education, 22*(1), 35–48.

Rahnema, M. (1992). Poverty. In W. Sachs (Ed.), *The development dictionary: A guide to knowledge as power* (pp. 158–176). Zed Books.

Rahnema, M. (2001). *Poverty*. Available: http://www.pudel.uni-bremen.de/pdf/majid2.pdf. Last accessed 28 June 2003.

Reason, P. (1994). *Participation in human inquiry*. Sage.

Rebera, R. (1997). Polarity or partnership? Retelling the story of Martha and Mary from Asian women's perspective (Luke 10: 38-42). *SEMEIA: An Experimental Journal for Biblical Criticism, 78*, 93–107.

Revill, G. (1993). Reading Rosehill: Community, identity and inner-city Derby. In M. Keith & S. Pile (Eds.), *Place and the politics of identity* (pp. 117–140).

Robinson, F. (1988). *Varieties of South Asian Islam*. Centre for Research in Ethnic Relations, University of Warwick.

Rogers, E. M. (1976). Communication and development – The passing of the Dominant Paradigm. In E. M. Rogers (Ed.), *Communication and development: Critical perspectives* (pp. 121–148). Sage.

Room, G. (1995). Poverty in Europe: Competing paradigms of analysis. *Policy and Politics, l23*(2), 103–113.

Rose, N. (1999). *Powers of freedom: Reframing political thought*. Cambridge University Press.

Rostow, W. (1960). *The stages of economic growth: A non-communist manifesto*. Cambridge University Press.

Ryff, C. D., & Singer, B. (1998). The contours of positive human health. *Psychological Inquiry, 9*, 1–28.

Sabat, M. N. (2002). Toward a visionary politics: Phenomenology, psychoanalytic feminism, and transcendence. In R. F. Groenhout (Ed.), *Philosophy, feminism, and faith* (p. 270). Indiana University Press.

Sachs, W. (1990). The archaeology of the development idea, *Interculture, Xxiii* (Issue, No 4), 2–37.

Saeed, S. (2009). Negotiating power: Community media, democracy, and the public sphere. *Development in Practice, 19*(4/5), 466–478.

Said, E. (1995). *Orientalism*. Penguin.

Samad, Y. (2004). Muslim youth in Britain: Ethnic to religious identity, Paper presented at the International Conference *Muslim Youth in Europe. Typologies of religious belonging and socio-cultural dynamics*, Edoardo Agnelli Centre for Comparative Religious Studies, Turin, 11th June 2004.

Sardar, Z. (1997). *Postmodernism and the other: The new imperialism of Western culture*. Pluto.

Sardar, Z. (2002). Islam resistance and reform. *New Internationalist [Online Version]*. http://www.newint.org/features/2002/05/01/keynote-islam-resistance-and-reform/. Date Accessed June 2002.

Sardar, Z., & Van Loon, B. (1999). *Introducing cultural studies*. Icon.

Sarup, M. (1988). *An introductory guide to post-structuralism and postmodernism* (2nd ed.). Hemel.

Sarwar, G. (1992). *Sex education: The Muslim perspective*. Muslim Educational Trust.

Saul, B., & Bryman, A. (Eds.). (2004). *Understanding research for social policy and practice: Themes, methods and approaches*. Policy Press.

Saunders, P., & Tsumori, K. (2002). Poor concepts: Social exclusion, poverty and the politics of guilt. *Policy, 18*(2), 32.

Sayyid, S. B. (1997). *A fundamental fear: Eurocentrism and the emergence of Islamism*. Zed Books.

Schiller, H. I. (1976). *Communication and cultural domination*. New York: International Arts and Sciences Press.

Schofield, V. (1996). *Kashmir in the crossfire*. London: I.B. Tauris.

Schramm, W. (1964). *Mass media and national development*. Stanford University Press.

Servaes, J. (1995). Development communication - For whom and for what? *Communication, 21*(I), 39–49.

Servaes, J. (1999). *Communication for development. One world, multiple cultures*. Hampton Press.

SEU. (1997). *Purpose, work priorities and working methods*. The Stationery Office.

SEU. (1998). *Truancy and school exclusion*. The Stationary Office.

SEU. (2000). *Minority ethnic issues in social exclusion and neighborhood renewal*. The Stationery Office.

SEU. (2001). *A new commitment to neighborhood renewal: National strategy action plan*. The Stationery Office.

Shah, S. (1998). A muddled maze: Reworking the routes. In K. Haw & S. Shah (Eds.), *Educating Muslim girls: Shifting discourses* (pp. 147–158). Open University Press.

Shannon, C., & Weaver, W. (1949). *A mathematical model of communication*. University of Illinois Press.

Shaw, A. (1988). *Pakistani community in Britain*. Blackwell.

Sheridan, A. (1980). *Micheal Foucault, the will to truth*. Tavistock.

Sheridan, L. P. (2006). Islamophobia pre– and post–September 11th, 2001. *Journal of Interpersonal Violence, 21*(3), 317–336. 10.1177/0886260505282885.

Silver, H. (1994). Social exclusion and social solidarity: Three paradigms. *International Labour Review, 133*, 531.

Skeggs, B. (1994). Situating the production of feminist ethnography. In M. Maynard & J. Purvis (Eds.), *Researching women's lives from a feminist perspective*. Taylor and Francis.

Skelton, T., & Allen, T. (1999). *Culture and global change* (T. Skelton & T. Allen, Eds.). Routledge.

Smaje, C. (1995). *Health, 'race' and ethnicity: Making sense of the evidence*. Kings Fund.

Smaje, C. (1996). The ethnic patterning of health: New directions for theory and research. *Sociology of Health and Illness, 18*(2), 139–171. https://doi.org/10.1111/1467-9566.ep10934605.

Smith, C. W. (1959). *Islam in modern history*. New American Library.

Smith, J. K. (1990). Alternative research paradigms and the problem of criteria. In E. Guba (Ed.), *The paradigm dialog* (pp. 167–187). Sage.

Smith, J. K. (1991). A methodology for twenty-first century sociology. *Social Forces, 70*, 1–17.

Smith, R. (1999). Medicine and the marginalised. *British Medical Journal, 18*(319), 1589–1590.

Smith, G. D. (Ed.). (2002). *Inequalities in health: The evidence presented to the independent inquiry into inequalities in health*. The Policy Press.

Smith, L., II. (1999). *Decolonizing methodologies: Research and indigenous peoples*. Zed Books.

Solmos, J., & Back, L. (1995). Marxism, racism and ethnicity. *American Behavioral Scientist, 38*(3), 407–420.

Sreberny-Mohammedi, A. (1996). Globalisation, communication and transnational civil society. In S. Braman & A. Sreberny-Mohammedi (Eds.). Hampton.

Stacey, J. (1988). Can there be a feminist ethnography? *Women's Studies International Forum, 11*(1), 21–27.

Stanfield, J. H., II. (1994). Ethnic modeling in qualitative research. In N. Denzin & Y. Lincoln (Eds.), *Handbook of qualitative research* (pp. 175–188). Sage.

Stanley, L., & Wise, S. (1993). *Breaking out again: Feminist ontology and epistemology*. Routledge.

Stappers, J., Olderaan, F., & de Wit, P. (1992). The Netherlands: The emergence of a new medium. In J. Jankowski, O. Prehn, & J. Stappers (Eds.), *The people's voice: Local radio and television in Europe*. John Libbey.

Statham, P. (1999). Political mobilisation by minorities in Britain: A negative feedback of 'race relations'? *Journal of Ethnic and Migration Studies, 25*(4), 597–626.
Stavenhagen, R. (1986). Ethno-development: A neglected dimension in development thinking. In R. Anthorpe & A. Kráhl (Eds.), *Development studies: Critique and renewal*. E J Brill.
Steeves, H. L. (1993). Creating imagined communities: Development communication and the challenge of feminism. *Journal of Communications, 43*(3), 218–229.
Stein, L. (1998). Democratic 'talk', access television and participatory political communication. *The Public, 5*(2), 21–34.
Stopforth, S., Kapadia, D., Nazroo, J., & Bécares, L. (2021). Ethnic inequalities in health in later life, 1993–2017: The persistence of health disadvantage over more than two decades. *Ageing and Society*, 1–29. https://doi.org/10.1017/S0144686X2100146X
Sue, S. (1999). Science, ethnicity, and bias: Where have we gone wrong? *American Psychologist, 54*(12), 1070–1077. https://doi.org/10.1037/0003-066X.54.12.1070
Sufyan, D. (2022). *British Muslims, ethnicity and health inequalities*. Edinburgh University Press.
Tandon, R. (1989). Participatory research and social transformation. *Convergence, 21*(2/3), 5–15. The American University. Available from: http://www.ourmedianet.org/papers/om2001/Atton.om2001.pdf (27 March, 2004).
Taylor, R. B. (1997). Social order and disorder of street blocks and neighborhoods: Ecology, microecology, and the systemic model of social disorganization. *Journal of Research in Crime and Delinquency, 34*(1), 113–155.
Tehranian, M. (1994). Communication and development. In D. Crowley & D. Mitchell (Eds.), *Communication theory today*. Polity Press.
Tipps, D. C. (1973). Modernisation theory and comparative study of societies: A critical perspective. *Comparative Studies in Society and History, 15*, 199–226.
Townsend, P. (1979). *Poverty in the United Kingdom*. Penguin.
Turner, B. S. (1993). *Religion and social theory*. London etc.: Sage.
Turner, B. S. (2003). Class, generation and Islamism: Towards a global sociology of political Islam. *The British Journal of Sociology, 54*(1), 139–147. https://doi.org/10.1080/0007131032000045941.
Turner, J. D. (1994). *An introduction to liberation theology*. Lanham, MD: University Press of America.
UNESCO. (1980). *Many voices, one world* (3rd ed.). Harmondsworth: Report by the International Commission for the Study of communication problems. UNESCO.
Unger, R. K. (1983). Through the looking glass: No Wonderland yet! (The reciprocal relationship between methodology and models of reality). *Psychology of Women Quarterly, 8*, 9–32.
Usher, R. (1996). A critique of the neglected epistemological assumptions of educational research. In D. Scott & R. Usher (Eds.), *Understanding educational research*. Routledge.
Valbuena, T. V. (1988). *Mahaweli Community Radio Project: An evaluation*. Asian Mass Communication Research and Information Centre.
Wahid, A. (2001). Islam, nonviolence and national transformation. In D. G. Paige, S. C. Anad, & S. Gilliathby (Eds.), *Islam and nonviolence* (pp. 53–57). Centre for Global Governance.
Wallerstein, I. (1974). *The modern world-system, vol. I: Capitalist agriculture and the origins of the European world-economy in the sixteenth century*. Academic Press.
Wallerstein, N. (1992). Powerlessness, empowerment and health: Implication for health promotion programs. *American Journal of Health Promotion., 6*(3), 197–205.
Wallerstein, N., & Freudenberg, N. (1998). Linking health promotion and social justice: A rationale and two case stories. *Health Education Research, 13*(3), 451–457.
Wallerstein N. B., & Duran, B. (2006, July). Using community-based participatory research to address health disparities. *Health Promot Pract, 7*(3), 312–323. https://doi.org/10.1177/1524839906289376. Epub 2006 Jun 7. PMID: 16760238.
Whitehead Margaret Andy Pennington Lois Orton Shilpa Nayak Mark Petticrew Amanda Sowden and Martin White. (2016). How Could Differences in 'Control Over Destiny' Lead to

Socio-Economic Inequalities in Health? A Synthesis of Theories and Pathways in the Living Environment. *Health and Place*, 51–61. https://doi.org/10.1016/j.healthplace.2016.02.002

Walsh, D. (2000). Doing ethnography. In C. Seale (Ed.), *Researching society and culture* (2nd ed., pp. 226–237). Sage.

Walsh, J., & Mcgrath, F. (2000). Identity, coping style, and health behaviour among first generation Irish immigrants in England. *Psychology and Health, 15*, 467–482.

Wang, G., & Dissanyake, W. (1984). Culture, Development and change: Some explorative observations. In G. Wang & W. Dissanayake (Eds.), *Continuity and change in communication systems* (pp. 3–20). Ablex.

Warburton, D. (Ed.). (1998). *Community and sustainable development: Participation in the future*. Earthscan Publications.

Wasko, J., & Mosco, V. (Eds.). (1992). *Democratic communications in the information age*. Garamond Press & Ablex.

Weedon, C. (1997). *Feminist practice and poststructuralist theory* (2nd ed.). Blackwel.

Weller, P., Feldman, A., & Purdam, K. (2001). *Religious discrimination in England and Wales*. Home Office Research Study 220. Home Office.

Werbner, P. (2002). *Imagined diasporas among Manchester Muslims: The cultural performance of transnational identity politics*. James Currey Publishers.

Werbner, P. (2005). The translocation of culture: 'Community cohesion' and the force of multiculturalism in history. *The Sociological Review, 54*(4), 745–768.

Werbner, P., & Modood, T. (1997). *Debating cultural hybridity*. Zed Books.

WGSG. (1997). *Feminist geographies: Explorations in diversity and difference*. Longman.

White, S. (1994). *Participatory communication: Working for change and development*. Sage.

Whitehead, M. (1987). *The health divide: Inequalities in health for the 1980s*. Health Education Council.

Wilkinson, R. (1996). *Unhealthy societies: The afflictions of inequality*. Routledge.

Wilkinson, R., & Marmot, M. (Eds.). (1998). *Social determinants of health: The solid facts*. Centre for Urban Health, World Health Organization.

Williams, D. R. (2012). Miles to go before we sleep: Racial inequities in health. *Journal of Health and Social Behavior, 53*(3), 279–95. http://www.jstor.org/stable/41725217.

Williams, R. (1976). *Blamming the victims*. Vintage Books.

Williams, R. A., Eley, S., Hunt, K., & Bhatt, S. (1997). Has psychological distress among British Asians been underestimated? A comparison of three measures in the West of Scotland population. *Ethnicity and Health, 1997*(2), 21–29.

WHO. (1986). Ottawa Charter for Health Promotion: First International Conference on Health Promotion: Ottawa, 21 November 1986: Who/HPR/HEP/95.1. S.l.: World Health Organization.

WHO. (1998). The Jakarta Declaration on health promotion in the 21st century. *Health Millions, 24*(1), 29–30, 35. PMID: 12348529.

Yates-Doerr, Emily. (2020). Reworking the social determinants of health: Responding to material-semiotic indeterminacy in public health interventions. *Medical Anthropology Quarterly, 34*(3), 378–397. https://doi.org/10.1111/maq.12586

Young, I. M. (1990a). The ideal of community and the politics of difference. In L. J. Nicholson (Ed.), *Feminism/Postmodernism* (pp. 300–323). Routledge.

Young, I. M. (1990b). *Justice and the politics of difference*. Princeton.

Young, S. (2001). *Poverty in Nottingham report*. Nottingham Observatory.

Zimmerman, Marc, A., & Rappaport, J. (1988). Citizen participation, perceived control, and psychological empowerment. *American Journal of Community Psychology, 16*(5), 725–750. https://doi.org/10.1007/bf00930023

Zweig, M. (1991). *Religion and economic justice*. Philadelphia: Temple University Press.

Index[1]

[1] Note: Page numbers followed by 'n' refer to notes.

F. Malik, *Addressing Health Inequalities through Community Media*,
https://doi.org/10.1007/978-3-031-35237-9